"The Mama Sutra .... the first months of parenthood. This book is an entertaining read for any parent dealing with newborn issues such as gas, constipation, fussiness, and sleeplessness."

—Blake Alban, MD, pediatrician, UCLA

"Whether you're a first-time parent or going for your second or third, you'll appreciate having *The Mama Sutra*—essentially a holistic baby coach—in the palm of your hand. It's light and fun—and most important, it works!"

—Jenna Dewan

"The feeling of helplessness as a new parent when you can't calm your fussy baby is gut-wrenching. Thanks to *The Mama Sutra*, you will be a hero in your little one's eyes."

—Chris Pegula, author of *Diaper Dude*

"No more frantic Googling needed! These tried-and-true practices presented in a lighthearted and straightforward way make *The Mama Sutra* a must for all parents. Happy farting!"   —Kate Albrecht and Joey Zehr, *Mr. Kate*

"Who knew there were so many ways to burp a baby?! Thanks to *The Mama Sutra*, first-time parents like us will be better equipped to face the sleepless nights to come."

—Ashley Iaconetti and Jared Haibon

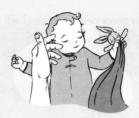

allie kingsley baker
and tony baker

ILLUSTRATIONS BY
Amy Jindra &
Nicholas Schlavensky

the
mama sutra

ANCIENT POSITIONS AND PRACTICES

TO SOOTHE THE MODERN BABY

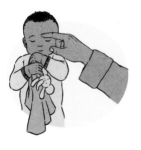

A TarcherPerigee Book

an imprint of Penguin Random House LLC
penguinrandomhouse.com

TarcherPerigee with tp colophon is a registered trademark of
Penguin Random House LLC.

Most TarcherPerigee books are available at special quantity discounts for bulk purchase for sales promotions, premiums, fund-raising, and educational needs. Special books or book excerpts also can be created to fit specific needs. For details, write:
SpecialMarkets@penguinrandomhouse.com.

Library of Congress Cataloging-in-Publication Data

Names: Baker, Allie Kingsley, author. | Baker, Tony (Screenwriter), author. |
Jindra, Amy, illustrator. | Schlavensky, Nicholas, illustrator.
Title: The mama sutra: ancient positions and practices to
soothe the modern baby / by Allie Kingsley Baker and Tony Baker;
illustrations by Amy Jindra & Nicholas Schlavensky
Description: [New York, New York]: TarcherPerigee, [2021]
Identifiers: LCCN 2020024986 (print) | LCCN 2020024987 (ebook) |
ISBN 9780593187623 (paperback) | ISBN 9780593187630 (ebook)
Subjects: LCSH: Infants—Care—Popular works. | Infants—Care—Handbooks,
manuals, etc. | Hatha yoga for infants.
Classification: LCC RJ61 .B17 2021 (print) | LCC RJ61 (ebook) | DDC 618.92/01—dc23
LC record available at https://lccn.loc.gov/2020024986
LC ebook record available at https://lccn.loc.gov/2020024987
p.   cm.

Printed in the United States of America
1st Printing

BOOK DESIGN BY KATY RIEGEL

For our daughter, Kingsley,

and her brother on the way.

And our first babies,

our niece and nephew, Henley and Cade.

the mama sutra

introduction

She was turning purple; we were turning green. Her screams amounted to "Help me, you incompetent fools!" She wasn't even nine pounds, but with her in our arms, we carried the weight of the world, because she had become our whole world. A world we thought we'd mapped out. Like everyone else, we read the parenting books. Okay, we read a lot of articles. All right, we *bought* a lot of books and skimmed a lot of articles on our phones. Who has time to read those things? Babies just eat, sleep, and poop, right? How tough could it be to manage that routine for something the size of an eggplant? But we weren't managing.

We stood over the changing table, anxiety sweating, while she flailed around in what was clearly record-setting agony for an eggplant. We had nothing to offer that she hadn't already declined. No other tools at our disposal. We were helpless, and that helplessness was the worst feeling either of us had ever experienced. We were helpless in the face of a fart.

Previously—we're talking a lifetime of observation here—farts were funny. Tony sneeze-farted in his fifth-grade English class while reading aloud *Huck Finn* and never lived it down. Allie (allegedly) sounded a foghorn the first night we slept together. Hilarious! But in this moment the laughter had gone silent and deadly. We were dealing with serious gas, seriously trapped in our newborn's belly. It wasn't funny at all.

Our article skimming had failed us, and in the dire immediacy of our baby's tortured tummy, picking up a book that weighed more than she did was not an option. We needed actions, not words. Over the next twenty-four hours, we gave her two different types of gripe water. We cycled through bottle brands and nipple flows. Out of desperation, we finally stuck a plastic tube lubed with coconut oil up her butt. And, sure, the plastic tube whistled as that little fucker of a fart found its way into the nursery, and absolutely there was a moment of relief shortly after.

But as the three of us lay in bed, avoiding eye contact, the consensus was obvious: There had to be a better way.

Not just a better way to relieve gas but better ways to help our baby in every circumstance. We wanted more options when the limited advice we'd found failed. We wanted to be experts in a variety of techniques to calm fussiness, to induce bowel movements, and to encourage better sleep. We didn't want to feel we had to resort to pumping our baby full of medication or jabbing her with foreign objects. We wanted to be *professional* parents.

As adults, when something goes awry, we don't jump to extremes to find quick relief. When our backs hurt, we stretch, get a massage, or see a chiropractor before asking the doctor for painkillers. If we're backed up, we drink water, eat a prune or two, and maybe invest in a Squatty Potty *before* downing a gallon of psyllium husk and sitting on an enema. Why shouldn't our babies get the same time and attention to detail and process we give ourselves?

Thus began our exploration of the broader world of infant care. We learned that knowing all the options was necessary because what works for Hazel won't necessarily sit well with Jacob. In discovering the diversity of theory and technique that's out there, we were able to adopt a more bespoke approach to tackling our baby's daily challenges.

And though we did ultimately find the information we sought, it was extremely challenging to come by. It was scattered all over those baby books and the Internet like crumbs from a smashed cake, and it was just as hard to gather together. Some of it came from conversations we had with top pediatricians, pediatric chiropractors and massage therapists, and world-renowned sleep experts. We found gems that amounted to a king's ransom, but each person had only two or three, and no two were alike. Our journey became less like a research project and more like a scavenger hunt. Put another way, there was a comprehensive multidisciplinary approach to baby care that existed but had yet to be collated into a single resource.

It got us thinking. Once upon a time, boxing and kung fu and jujitsu were all separate martial arts. Then someone decided they should be pitted against each other to see which was the best. Through that competition, the glorious art form known as mixed martial arts, or MMA, was born, taking what worked best from all the disparate martial arts traditions of the world.

Similarly, our journey led us to uncover a trove of internationally and historically vetted traditions—a variety of means, both modern and ancient, by which we could attempt to solve our baby's woes. Best of all, many of them worked! They worked for our baby, and they worked for us. No longer were we without recourse. The slack-jawed, incompetent losers our baby was born to gave way to the finely tuned champions who write this now. The feeling of helplessness we had in the face of her distress was conquered, and we found we had assembled our own parenting style.

The MAMA Sutra is:

Mixed—*This approach is a combination of the best techniques from many disciplines.*

Adaptive—*You will learn to take note of your baby's cues and figure out which techniques work for them. This will be an evolving process as they grow and their needs change.*

Medicinal—*Everything is aimed at providing aid and/ or relief.*

Attentive—*This is what your baby needs more than*

anything in order to put the approaches here into best practice. You must commit to attending to and being attentive to your baby's needs.

Your baby is trying to communicate with you, and she is using a language that's completely her own. You must learn to listen to it. Discovering this was the landmark unanticipated benefit to our hunt. Learning the nuances of our baby's language was both enlightening and rewarding. It not only made us more capable and confident in our ability to parent, it made us baby whisperers. We could decipher the difference between her clenched fart fists, and her constipated double-leg kick, and her I-need-to-go-the-fuck-to-sleep eye rub. We had learned to immediately offer her the remedy she desired while forging a stronger bond through caring touch and loving communication. It's in this spirit that we encourage you to also use these techniques. You will find an untapped joy in being able to recognize and respond to your little one's one-of-a-kind requests.

We'll get a bit playful when discussing and drawing upon the other sutras, but we have the utmost respect for those sacred traditions. The Mama Sutra modernizes the ancient art of holistic healing through positions, holds, massage, stretches, stimuli, and more. As you explore the contents of this book and put its methods into practice, your understanding of your baby's particular cues will grow, and you will become an expert on your own child.

Not only that, you have almost completed the wordiest section in this book. When our baby was having gas issues, we didn't have time or energy to read a hundred pages on how gas is made. We wanted to flip to the page that read, *Baby won't sleep? Try this! The Mama Sutra* does just that. It is an easily digestible (pun intended) quick-reference guide. We know what it is like to be exhausted beyond measure and stressed to the point of breaking. There isn't room for anything but doing. We're right there with you and offer this as an accessible helping hand in those most trying of moments.

We're repeating ourselves a bit but feel it's worth noting one more time: It's important to remember that when you are up against your baby's upset and discomfort, there is no one-size-fits-all cure. We present a multitude of possible solutions to try, with the idea that only you can discover which ones work best for your babe. Additionally, you might find that one of these techniques works exceptionally well at three months, but just weeks later, a different way proves superior.

Our babies are our most awesome responsibility. And while responding to their cues comes naturally, having the ability to respond effectively takes some getting-to-know-you trial and error. Cycling through these techniques empowered us. It gave us the "able" part we lacked in wanting to be response-able parents. If your baby is lucky enough not to have any of the difficulties or discomforts addressed in this book, we encourage you to still work your way through the pages. These positions and movements are a great opportunity for you to interact, bond with, and stimulate your little one.

Without further delay, the Mama Sutra.

the gas guru

Imagine being stuck in the bowels of a sinking ship, tumbling through the depths toward the ocean floor. The power is out, and it's pitch-black. You know you've got to get out of there, but you have no idea which way is up and which way is down. This is the life experience of your baby's trapped gas. It wants out. It's running the hallways of her intestines, banging against the walls while screaming. If only someone would help it find its way to the surface! Meanwhile, the ship is in chaos. The alarm is at full volume. The sprinkler system has been triggered. The flares are in the air. Oh, and by the way, you're the captain.

This chapter is about navigating bubbles out of the SS *Flatulator* by gently tilting, rocking, and otherwise manipulating the ship, a.k.a. your baby.

Gas can originate in one of two ways: swallowing air or having trouble digesting food. Consider that your baby spent the first nine months of existence underwater (not breathing air) and taking in nutrition from a tube in their belly button (not swallowing or digesting). Guess what happens when you pop the sack and stick a nipple in her mouth? She gets gassy. Life for all would be smoother sailing if only those bubbles would become cute toots. But too often they remain in your baby's tummy, causing pain, irritation, and fussiness.

You must *actively* encourage this little person to fart, and fart often. Try to keep in mind that the adjustment she is making to her new environment is challenging.

On average, babies pass gas thirteen to twenty-one times a day. (If you are not shocked by this because you are on a similar schedule, we encourage you to seek out a dietician or perhaps medical help.) The moral of that statistic is not to worry if it sounds like there's a high school band marching through your baby's diaper. Your baby *should be* abnormally gassy when compared to anything in the universe other than stars, cars . . . or other babies.

Like an SUV, babies are gas-guzzlers from the minute they're born. Within seconds of arrival they're swallowing air as they scream for the first time. They'll ingest even more air as they cry, laugh, eat, and adjust to their new world. Other gas influencers include improper feeding positions, intolerance to different foods, and food allergies. With that in mind, the movements in this section work best when in conjunction with other adjustments. For example, if you're bottle-feeding, consider an anti-gas variety or a slow-flow nipple so your babe swallows less air when he eats. Or you might want to talk to your doctor about changing formula. Or, if you're breastfeeding, the foods you're eating might not agree with his belly. A lactation consultant can also help with positioning and latch. Sometimes the situation does call for anti-gas drops or other medicines, and if it comes to that, that's okay, too.

how to tell if your baby has gas

Unpassed gas is a pain in the ass. In addition to crying—which accompanies pretty much anything that might be bothering your baby—you'll recognize the specific signs of gas if you know what to look for. They include a hard-to-the-touch or distended belly, the clenching of their fists, and the arching of their back.

struggling turtle

If you ask someone how to relieve your baby's abdominal distension, this technique is likely the first suggestion you'll get. So in our quest to alleviate gas, this is where the guru's journey begins. This position draws its name from the image it conjures: a tiny creature, supine on its back, and in distress. However, unlike the assistance you might offer an actual turtle, the goal here is not to roll your baby over onto all fours. Instead, you're going to be using his knees to create a delicate pulsating pressure on his tummy. This should make baby's gas feel sufficiently uncomfortable in its current home and start looking to move. In addition to the helpful pressure created by pumping their legs, you're stimulating circulation and blood flow, which encourages their body's natural response system to react faster.

1. Start with your baby on their back, on a flat and safe surface.
2. With a light grip on both of his ankles, lift and

delicately bounce his bootie up and down. This creates a gentle pressure in his abdomen.

3. Alternate bending each knee toward his stomach as if he's riding a bicycle. Each bend presses into the tummy and then extends all the way straight to get a full range of motion.

Practice this sequence until your babe's belly is relieved or as long as he's happy doing so.

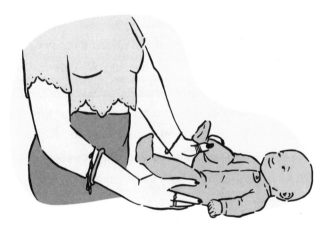

pouch pose

Unlike our marsupial friends, if we want to carry our kids around in a stomach pouch, we have to buy a sling or carrier. However, to execute this pose, all you need is a comfortable place to sit and two hands. This position can be helpful in combating GERD (gastroesophageal reflux disease, of which the most common sign for babies is frequent vomiting) and is even more effective against milder, more common forms of acid reflux.

With acid reflux, the pain and discomfort come from the acid backing up into our esophagus. This is made worse when we lie down or tilt back, which is how your little one spends most of her time. If your baby is prone to reflux, then you might want to perfect Pouch Pose for a double whammy of relieving gas and keeping the acid down. It also engages baby's core muscles, which will expedite the extradition while transferring uncomfortable pressure to less sensitive areas. Additionally, while in Pouch Pose they're pressed against your body and close to your heart, leading to feelings of comfort and contentment—for you both.

Take a seat somewhere stable and safe.

1. Start with your baby on your lap, facing away
   from you.
2. Place one hand under her belly and the other hand
   beneath her chest. You should be safely supporting
   her as you tilt her forward at a forty-five-degree angle
   and let her rest in that position. If your baby is unable
   to support her head, rather than placing one hand on
   her chest, use it to support her chin and neck.

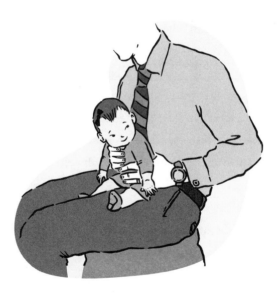

diving dolphin

This is not a position you want to include in your repertoire until baby has enough strength to hold her head up on her own, around four to six months. Once they hit that milestone, it's time to bring a bit of the beach into your living room. Think beach ball. Think dolphins.

You don't have to use an actual beach ball; yoga or balance balls work as well. You just want a ball that's big enough that baby arches over it in the same approximate shape as a dolphin when diving. It should be firmly inflated so that it supports their weight.

This is a fun activity even if baby isn't struggling with gas. Ours laughs hysterically every time we play this game. In fact, we don't suggest this technique when your baby is crying full throttle. Instead, make it a fun activity when they're already happy and it will help in more ways than one.

1. With the support of *both* your hands, lay your baby tummy down over the top of a large ball. Hopefully

it goes without saying, but do not ever let go of your baby when practicing this position.

2. Using his own body weight (without pressing down or adding pressure), and with both hands on the baby, roll him back and forth, side to side. You should only roll him a few inches each way, never tilting him downward. Stick with subtle moves to softly compress the belly area.

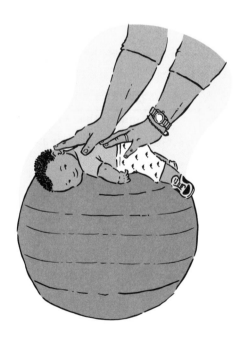

swaying cobra

You will not need a flute or magical powers to charm your baby. Let's focus on the enchanted cobra here: their head aloft and flared, swaying back and forth while their belly slithers around on the ground, attempting to steady the extra weight. That Swaying Cobra is what we want to see from your baby at tummy time. When your baby is forced to lift her head and look around, it helps her achieve a number of other physical milestones. Keeping it up is the precursor to rolling over, crawling, and eventually walking. It aids in developing muscles throughout the upper body. Another benefit of tummy time? Gas relief!

The goal is to get fifteen to twenty minutes of tummy time a day; for fussy babies, they say that five minutes at a time up to three times a day will suffice. It's totally normal if at first your baby fights you on being belly down, but over time they'll learn to love this exploratory position. It's worth mentioning that the only time for tummy time is while the baby is awake and under your watchful eye.

1. After feeding and burping, place your babe belly down on a soft, flat surface, over a Boppy pillow, or in your lap.

2. Keep them engaged with colorful play mats, toys with various textures, or entertaining lights.

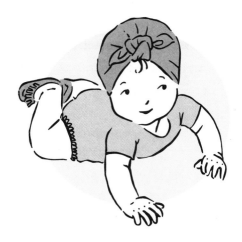

lucky rabbit

In many cultures, carrying a rabbit's foot is good luck. Being fans of all beings with fur, we prefer an animal-friendly approach. Acupressure massage stimulates circulation and energy flow using specific pressure points tied to certain areas of the body. The reflux points for gas are located in the arch and heel of your baby's foot. And let's be honest, who doesn't appreciate a foot massage? Rubbing your baby's foot with your thumb won't likely bring great fortune or a bountiful harvest (or maybe it will?), but it will without question encourage gas relief.

Your touch should be stronger than a tickle or stroke but delicate enough not to bust a peeled hard-boiled egg.

For this topic, we consulted Dr. Amy Albright, a doctor of acupuncture and Chinese medicine (DACM), who reminded us that it's important to be tender with your touch and use your best judgment in applying loving and light pressure for no more than fifteen minutes per day.

1. Apply slight pressure by rubbing your thumb in circular motions across the arch and mid-foot.
2. Next, make your way to the heel area, this time moving it spot to spot around the heel and applying slight pressure instead of sweeping motions.
3. Hold each pressure point for about fifteen seconds.
4. Repeat steps 1 and 2 three times on each foot.

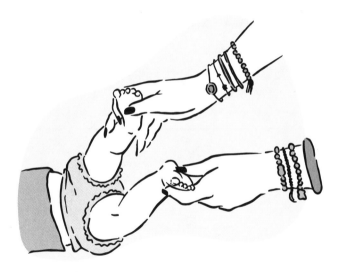

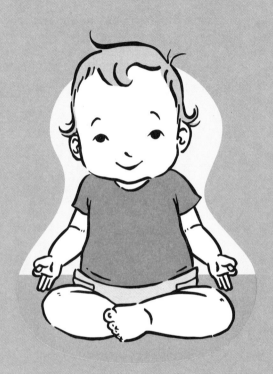

the burping buddha

It had been forever since we'd left the house. At least it felt that way. More specifically, it had been months since we had gone out for anything recreational, or did anything at all without our beautiful baby girl. Other couples we knew spun yarns about their glorious weekly date nights—vital, they said, to maintain a healthy marriage and relationship; an absolute necessity to retaining your sanity.

Those were the people who had help. If it wasn't a nanny, it was grandparents or aunts and uncles just a stone's throw away. But we were pretty much on our own, geographically speaking. We didn't yet have a reliable babysitter. No family nearby. No trustworthy assistance of any kind.

About a month into our baby-hibernation, Allie's

mother, Susan, came down from Seattle to stay with us for a weekend that happened to coincide with a friend's fortieth birthday party. The idea of getting gussied up and hitting the town was an opportunity we couldn't pass up.

Susan was more than thrilled to give us a few hours to live out our long-lost fantasies of being as sexy and social as we once were. We showed Grandma the necessities: the bottle warmer, baby's favorite swaddle, how to work the swing. Last but not least, a reminder to give our girl good burps throughout every feeding. Otherwise, she'd fill up like a balloon and hurt so badly that it would hurt you.

We got in the car and drove an hour and a half up the Pacific Coast Highway. We arrived at our favorite restaurant in Malibu, where we'd spent many a romantic eve and just so happened to be the location of our friend's shindig.

We didn't even sit together. We were so thrilled to see anyone other than each other, we spent the first part of our "date night" at separate tables catching up with the friends who forgivably may have assumed we had gone into witness protection. Surrounded by belly dancers, stuffing our faces with braised lamb and baklava, we whooped it up— for about twenty minutes.

The phone rang. It was Allie's mom on FaceTime. In the background, our daughter was screaming the unmistakable sound of gas pain. And Grandma was visibly flustered, not knowing what to do. "Burp her!" Allie hollered over the live band. Her mom put the phone down, and we watched as she put the baby over her shoulder and, with all the ferocity of a cotton ball hitting the ground, pat our daughter on the back. "No, Mom—harder! You need to give her a good whack!" Grandma's phone flipped over and disconnected. Allie started crying. Our friends, seasoned parents, served up a decent dose of first-time mom shame. *She's not going to die from gas. You're hormonal. Just wait until she starts eating solids.* We took a deep breath. They were right. She wasn't in harm's way. It was just gas, for crying out loud.

The phone rang again. This time Grandma was crying. "I think you should come home." We ripped back down the PCH, threading from lane to lane. "Move it, people! Our baby has to burp, dammit!"

Much of an infant's physical discomfort can stem from ineffective burping techniques. The classic over-the-shoulder position sometimes works, so Allie's mom wasn't wrong in trying it, but she wasn't doing it correctly. If firmly patting the baby was making Grandma uncomfortable, there is a plethora of positions to release their inner bullfrog, many of them more effective anyway.

The first few months will at times make you feel like a worker on an assembly line. It's just a long, repetitive chain of feeding and burping. This doesn't go on as long as it'll feel in the moment, but it's true what they say: The days are slow and the months are fast. (You'll miss it when she's cramming peas into the impossible-to-clean crevices of her high chair.)

While burping a baby is more art than science, there are some guidelines you can keep in mind. If you've been swatting your baby on the back for two, three, or four minutes and nothing is happening, it might be that you need to adjust your technique. However, it also might be that no matter what you do, the baby can't get the burp out. Taking that a step further, it also might be because the baby doesn't *have* to burp. (And, of course, if your little one is very upset and you're questioning whether they need medical attention, always call the pediatrician. That's what they're there for! We used to feel bad about calling the after-hours number, but that quickly passed. This is why they're paid the big bucks.) If a baby is fussy after feeding, it might just be that they need to be burped. As a general rule of thumb, once a little one can sit up on their own, they no longer need you to burp them.

Until such time, we give you the Burping Buddha. Nirvana is the ultimate goal of Buddhism. Ridding your baby of unwanted gas is the ultimate goal of new parenthood. We find no irony in that the literal meaning of the term *nirvana* is "to blow out."

bottles and nipples can make a big difference

If you're bottle-feeding, don't hold back when it comes to investing in a variety of bottle styles and nipple sizes. There are bottles specifically designed to reduce air intake during feedings and nipples with different flow speeds. We discovered we were not alone in that many babies cycle through a bunch of brands before finding the right one. Some stores even offer a "bottle box" with an assortment from some of the most popular brands, and friendly parents are often more than happy to let you test out their collections, too.

grandma's go-to

While this position has become the gold standard in belches, it's surprising that so many people (including us, at first) get it wrong. With this classic, the devil is in the details.

There are three elements you'll want to focus on:

1. The position of your shoulder to baby's torso.
2. The location on baby's back where you are patting.
3. And the amount of gumption applied to said patting.

When perfecting execution on all three, think in terms of micro-adjustments. Your baby is tiny, and so, too, is the target area. If your shoulder isn't slightly pressed into your babe's midsection, you won't bring about the best burp. If you tap too softly (we're looking at you, Nana Susan), the baby will not even notice you're there.

Position: Hold the baby on your chest, facing you, with one arm tucked under his bottom. If Mom's holding the babe, place his belly over your breast. This extra cushion adds a light pressure to his tummy, encouraging gas release! For dads (or moms with less cushion for the pushin'), bring the baby up higher so his belly is resting on your shoulder. This works for the same reason. Note: Do not bounce the baby if you are using your breast or shoulder for support; too much pressure could do more harm than good.

Patting: Be sure to slightly cup your hand, as it's gentler than a flat hand. Begin patting between the shoulder blades and make your way up, then down. After five to ten pats, give your baby's back a few soothing circular rubs and then return to patting.

For many babies, patting simply doesn't do the trick. Stick with rubbing instead. Circles, up and down, back and forth. When you find the spot, everyone will be happy.

drunk monk

Did you know that monks invented beer? It's true! They were the first to use hops in the fermentation process. As most of us *do* know, consumption of too much beer can lead to a loss of equilibrium resulting in tottering around the room in circles. Like a drunk monk, this technique takes your baby for a burp-inducing spin. It requires no patting at all, and therefore there's less guesswork. It works instead by stimulating your baby's core muscles, which in turn works the gas out. You are going to help him execute this motion by sitting him on your lap, with his hips stationary, while you slowly and carefully rotate his upper body.

1. Sit your little one down on your lap; one leg will do.
2. For younger babies who cannot support their head, place one of your hands under his chin to support the front of his head and your other hand on the back of his head and neck to support his body and skull. For older babies who can support their head, place one hand on their chest and the other on their

back. Once you feel that your baby is completely supported and secure, move on to the next step.

3. Slowly—no, really, *slowly*—circle your baby's torso while keeping their bottom firmly planted on your thigh. If your baby reacts well to this move, you should get some solid burps out!

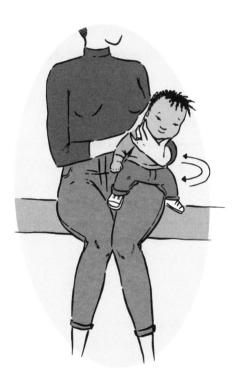

a cute asana

The asana was the original yoga pose: a comfortable seat for long periods of meditation—at least that's what we've heard. If this is true, it makes sense that the practice of yoga would need to expand to include other positions, because it's hard to get someone to put down thirty bucks for a one-hour class in learning how to sit.

The asana we recommend for helping your baby burp won't take an hour to perfect, much less execute. It is centered around a steady and comfortable position both for you and for baby, although baby will be more relaxed since you will be providing all of the necessary support and stimulation. Easing your baby into a Cute Asana should help him relax both body and mind, facilitating the easy release of a burp.

Think Pouch Pose, but for infants who cannot yet support their own head.

1. Start by finding a comfortable place for yourself to sit.
2. Sit your baby on your lap, facing away from you.

3. With your forearm supporting his torso and your thumb and forefinger underneath the jawline, supporting his head, lean him forward to a forty-five-degree angle until his full weight is supported.

4. Lightly pat and rub your baby's back between his shoulder blades until reflux nirvana is achieved.

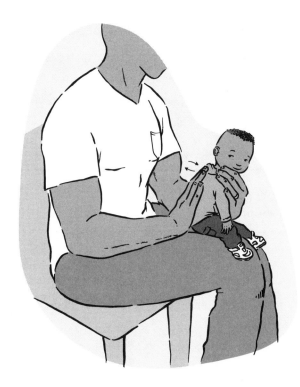

bowing belcher

Prostration is *not* a male gland, and this position *does not* require any sort of intrusive examination for Dad. Instead, prostration is a gesture used in many religious practices to show reverence. Simply imagined, it's a bow—sometimes a full bow that stretches one's entire body across the floor. Here, your lap will serve as baby's floor, and the reverence you offer is to the expulsion of internal discord.

Your baby will likely attempt to lift her head or avert her eyes. For our particular brand of deference, this is not a sign of disrespect. In fact, it's perfectly welcome, as it means your babe is strengthening her neck and back muscles. Allow your baby just enough range of motion to attempt to lift her head, without ever removing support completely.

1. Lay your baby across your lap. Align the strongest part of your thigh with their belly to offer a slight pressure.
2. Use your hand to support her head and neck by placing it beneath her jawline.

3. Alternate between lovingly patting and rubbing your baby between her shoulders and toward her upper back.

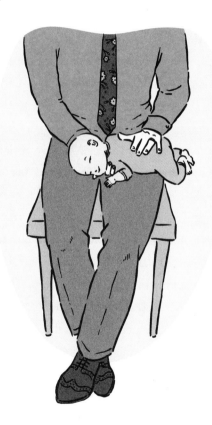

after chakras

While, traditionally speaking, there is no burp chakra, if there were, this technique might move energy through it. This one works best with a balance ball, a couch cushion with a bit of spring, or even the edge of your mattress, because you are going to be bouncing. We're working with the old adage of *what goes up must come down*—and what goes down sometimes comes up. When we get tense emotionally, we tighten ourselves physically, and the same goes for the littles. If you're wound up, that makes it tough to do things like sleep, poop, and burp. This move packs in a one-two punch in that it soothes your honey by smoothly bouncing (again employing womb-like movements) while patting to encourage the belch.

This is a variation on Grandma's Go-To, sans pressure on the belly, and is especially helpful for colicky babies who love constant movement and prefer to be bounced.

1. Hold your baby close to your chest, with one hand on their rear and the other supporting their neck and head.

2. Securely sit on your exercise ball (or couch or mattress or other bouncy thing) and gingerly bounce up and down while giving your baby a solid pat or rub.

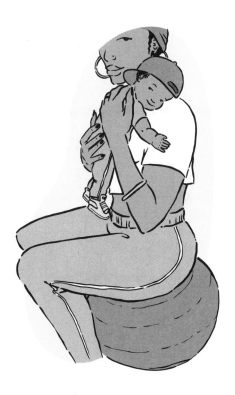

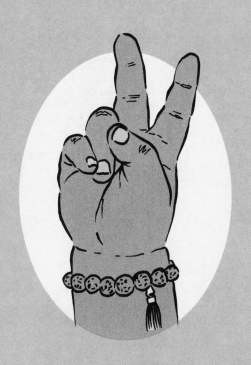

the sh*tting shaman

Time does not actually exist, at least not in the way we sometimes think about it as this invisible, unalterable, compelling force. Time is just a measure of movement. Humans invented the concept to track the sun, the moon, the stars, and our own planet. Think of it this way: Time doesn't make the world go around—the world makes time by going around. We use time as a way to plan and track our day-to-day progress as we attempt to grow, to achieve, to enjoy, to make the most of our movement through life. This is why, when your baby is stuck on a movement, time stands still.

Turds are like people. You're probably thinking, "Some people are like turds, too," and you're right, but that's beside the point. What we mean is, turds, like people, aspire to use their journey through life to reshape themselves—to emerge, if you will, from an amorphous beginning into a self-molded, well-defined presence. And just like people, sometimes in order to achieve this transformation, a turd requires the proper mentorship. They need an expert, a guide, a shaman, if you will, to reach their full potential. By assuming this role yourself, you can help turds of all kinds find their path. You can clear hurdles from their road and, in moments of darkness, light the way.

The journey is complicated to start because your baby has a brand-new digestive system, as well as a number of other brand-new physiological networks—networks that it is going to spend the rest of its existence coordinating with. If your company has ever tried to implement new software for the sake of streamlining operations, you know what a challenge this can be, and that's for a team of (mostly) competent adults. Now, this proverbial software is working together inside your baby using just-out-of-the-box tools. You can't change this, but you can make the work environment as conducive to success as possible. That's why a big part of training turds to fulfill their turdestiny comes from establishing a proper environment, which may simply mean adequate hydration or dietary changes.

Close your eyes and imagine that you, the adult, are lying flat on your back and shitting. Be honest. Do you think this is an easy, enjoyable way to unload? It is no different for your little one. Furthermore, if you ate six full meals a day, then spent most of the day asleep and your waking hours on your back, how effective do you think your system would be at processing those meals for energy and relieving waste? In addition to the positions in this section, you'll also find physical activities you can do with your new best friend, which will stimulate circulation, induce certain hormonal responses, and spur their immune system so they get all those inner workings up to speed.

After this chapter, you yourself will be a shitting shaman worthy of ceremonial dance.

froggy style

This Froggy Style squat is our number one go-to for releasing poop into the wild. Inspired by the ever popular Squatty Potty (shout-out!), the squat works for a number of reasons. Basically, at this angle, the rectal canal opens up, allowing for less strain and an easier, more productive poop.

1. Tuck her legs upward and out like a frog perched on a log. This position gives poop an easy way out. Let gravity work for your baby.
2. Hold the froggy pose for six seconds before lifting your baby up and giving those legs a stretch. Repeat this slow-motion hopping action until you hear a diaper croak.

NOTE: We sometimes hold our backed-up baby over the shoulder and froggy her legs to give her an abdominal assist.

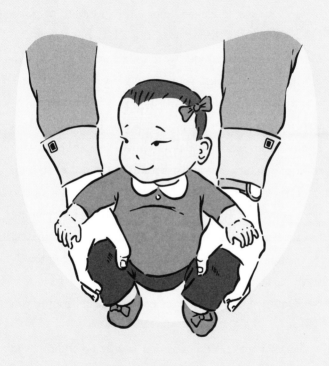

spraying mantis

When it comes to clogged pipes, this position, inspired by the porcelain throne, gets the job done. It was the most successful technique we found for our daughter. The dip in the hips relaxes your infant's lower half and gives gravity a hand, while aligning the colon with the small intestine, allowing for an unobstructed elimination. As a bonus, this position creates a roomy pocket in the diaper, minimizing blowouts and other unsightly messes.

The other great thing about this pose is that it can be done anywhere. If you notice that your baby is struggling to squeeze out a number two, all you need is a safe surface. At the pharmacy? Find a shelf, slide a row of paper towels to the side, and let your baby's bottom hang for a few. Stuck at the DMV? The back of the chair in front of you makes for a handy assist.

Please note that this position is only for infants who can support their own head.

1. With your baby facing away from you, place both of your hands beneath her armpits.

2. Rest her heels atop a safe surface; the knees should bend over the edge.
3. Dip her bottom slightly below knee level.
4. Hold this pose as long as your baby is happy and comfortable or until she's unloosed the caboose.

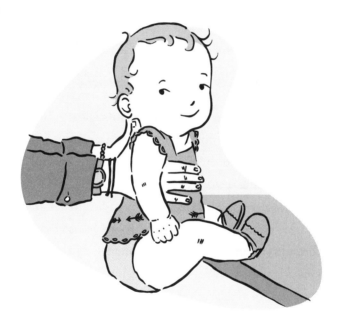

massaging for poop

(Not to be confused with a poop massage, which is highly unsanitary as well as illegal in most states)

It would be at best rude and at worst a cause for litigation for an adult to take a dump during a massage. For a baby, however, no such etiquette exists—and, honestly, it's pretty much the goal. We're not saying that if you massage your baby in the manners we are about to suggest, she will evacuate her bowels on cue. But it's a reasonable possibility. It's an even more reasonable possibility for this to occur shortly after.

Studies have shown that infant massage can strengthen the bond between parent and baby, promote faster weight gain, and encourage relaxation of parent and baby. Additionally, massage decreases the amount of the stress hormone cortisol in the body, which leads babies who receive regular massage to deeper and longer periods of sleep.

Massage also helps decrease discomfort from gas and colic and eases constipation. It can help with teething pains and stuffy noses, too. When you massage your babe, you're supporting their muscle tone, stimulating circulation, and boosting their nervous, brain, and immune systems—what the pros refer to as IRRS: interaction, relaxation, relief, and stimulation. All that aside, for our purposes we will be focusing on how you can rub your little one in a righteous effort to liquidate their assets.

Why Does Massage Make Baby Poop?

Massage is relaxing and it stimulates both the circulatory and digestive systems, much like a morning cup of coffee does for you. Since mixing java in with the baba is bad for baby, we need to accomplish these goals another way. We sought advice from Melanie Wattles, a Certified Infant Massage Instructor and the owner of Baby Strokes, an organization for teaching pediatric massage, who has over twenty-five years of pediatric and neonatal nursing experience. Here's what she told us.

Your baby's digestive system is brand-new and has no idea what it's doing. Remember, she used to eat through a cord attached to that cute little belly button. This whole swallowing thing is new, and babies struggle with that. So, too, do they struggle with the processing and expulsion side of things. Your fingers can provide guidance, a road map or GPS, if you will, for those moments when baby's digestion gets confused between which way is up and which way is down, or if it just gets lazy and decides to stop moving altogether. These techniques are actually massaging the digestive tract, softening the contents and moving things along.

When Is the Right Time to Massage?

Imagine receiving a deep tissue massage immediately after destroying a full bowl of spaghetti. Gross, right? Don't start poking and prodding after a meal. Or before one, for that matter. Wait until they've fully digested their milk and are in a Zen mood.

For babies who spit up or have reflux, keep them upright during massage by using a Boppy pillow or your legs for support.

Melanie says waiting about forty-five minutes after eating is a good guideline. She encourages any massage for gas, colic, or tummy to be done at diaper changes if the baby is having symptoms, or right before a bath. Massage for sleep can be done whenever it suits the parent and baby.

Relaxation massages, unlike the digestion ones, can be done when the baby is fussy or before a nap or bedtime.

How Do I Set the Mood?

Baby shouldn't be dressed for this, but that's not a hard rule. It's your baby's choice, really. For very fussy babies, it's okay to massage over their clothes. Since nobody wants to strip down and get a massage in a refrigerator, keep the room temperature around seventy-five degrees. If you want to take things up a notch (do it!), lay your babe on a warm towel from the dryer. Doesn't that sound divine? (Allie wishes someone would do this for her. Ahem, Tony.)

Dim the lights, pull the shades, and light a candle, or do whatever you have to do to make it dark and cozy. Cortisol, the stress hormone, responds to light, and we are looking to decrease the level of cortisol in order to say goodbye to tension in baby. If baby is holding tension in her body, you can bet on what else she's holding on to.

Turn off your phone. Wait! Please don't throw the book out the window! We know how terrifying the thought of disconnecting can be—you might miss the next six-pack selfie from your childless friend—but take heart: Babies don't have any interest in an hour-long massage. Five to ten minutes is all you need. Will it be a hard ten minutes? Of course. But being good parents is about knowing when to make sacrifices. Massaging for poop is one such time. This needs to be an uninterrupted communal activity.

Our infant massage therapist plays lullaby music or soothing sounds to set the mood, but as the baby grows and you want a more playful vibe, you can jam to nursery rhymes and sing to your baby.

A Word on Oils

Using the right kind of oil will make everything go smoother, and smooth moves is what we are aiming for. Oils prevent friction burns and allow your strokes to glide. So what is the "right kind" of oil? Well, you need to make sure that whatever you're using isn't in any way toxic, as it will be absorbed by your babe's skin. The guidelines are easy enough: Use only natural, clean, unscented oils. A rule of thumb is to ask yourself: Would I eat this on my salad? Or, better yet, is it okay if this goes into my baby's mouth? Because it almost certainly will. We like to use food-grade cold-pressed organic oils like almond, apricot, sunflower, safflower, or grapeseed.

If you are a fan of essential oils like lavender or chamomile, which are soothing and calming, our expert suggests using them in the diffuser or room spray—not on your babe's body. They're just too concentrated and intense. Besides, it promotes bonding for your little one to smell you as opposed to scented oils. If you really *must* use one, add a few drops to one of the carrier oils above.

Before you get started, warm your hands and the oil by rubbing them together.

> In Chinese medicine, strokes that go upward toward the heart are more stimulating and downward away from the heart are more relaxing. Try both, and then observe your baby to learn what he likes best and finds relaxing.

The International Association of Infant Massage (IAIM) stresses the importance of asking your baby permission to massage them. At first, we were like, "Excuse me, what?" But it makes sense. It is their body, of course, and they deserve as much respect as any of us. And since they can't respond with, "Yeah, sure—Swedish style on the glutes," their communication cues will let you know if they're into it. For example, if your baby responds by becoming still, smiling, cooing, gazing at you, and seeming happy and content, that indicates they're in the right mood for a rubdown. If they start fussing, twitching, clenching their fists, or kicking, this might not be the most opportune moment.

So, before you get started, make eye contact and ask, "May I give you a massage?" If they give you a sunny response, begin by tenderly running your warmed hands over their body from shoulders to heels.

Anything Else?

Yes. Keep in mind that massage is not *just* a means to your baby's end. You should be enjoying it as much as your baby does. This is a chance for the two of you to do something together. Regular practice will promote bonding, trust, and feelings of love. Make eye contact while sharing this sweet ritual, and pay close attention to your baby's nonverbal cues. Watch their reactions to each movement. If they don't like something, stop what you're doing and either brake for snuggles or switch it up.

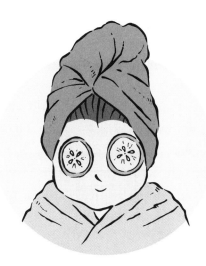

water wheel

These hand-over-hand strokes, which mimic a water wheel, are a pleasant yet effective way to get things moving. Start with your baby on their back, as always on a safe, flat surface.

1. Place your hands pinky-side down, palms facing you.
2. Place one hand under your baby's rib cage and scoop down his abdomen, stopping at the top of his diaper line.
3. Repeat with the other hand. Alternate sides.
4. Your touch should be gentle and fluid. Your baby's skin should move slightly in response but not pull.

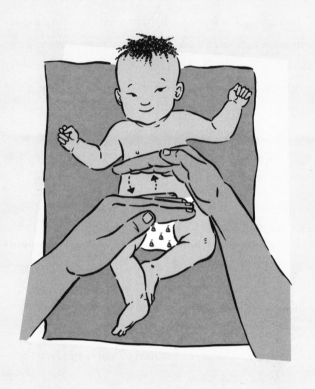

i love you

These strokes trace your baby's colon, encouraging elimination and relaxation. If someone massages my colon they'd better say "I love you" and buy me dinner—but you're basically doing both of those things on the reg with your munchkin, so it's cool.

You're going to trace an *I* down the left side of your baby's abdomen—the descending colon—followed by an upside-down *L* and then an upside-down *U*.

1. Use your forefinger and middle finger to draw the letter *I* down the left side of her tummy (your right).

2. Then draw an upside-down *L* going across the top of her tummy (left to right) and winding down again where the colon descends.

3. Draw an upside-down *U* up the ascending colon on her left side and back down on the right along the descending colon.

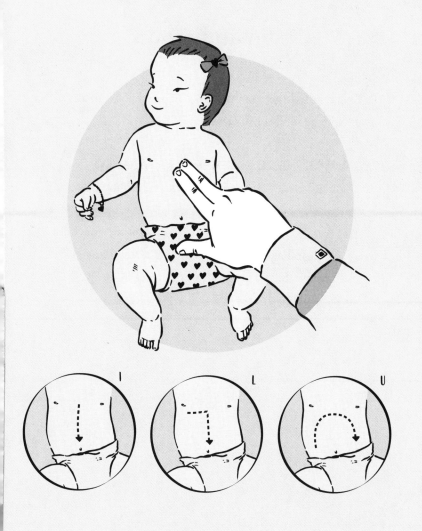

sun and moon

This celestial-themed massage is widely known to alleviate both gas and constipation.

1. With your left hand, slowly and continuously draw a full circle—the "sun"—clockwise around the whole of your baby's belly.

2. As your left hand reaches 12:00 and moves toward 6:00, follow it with your right hand, simultaneously tracing the shape of a crescent moon.

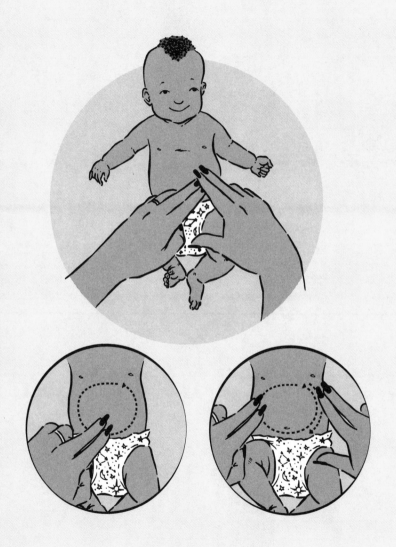

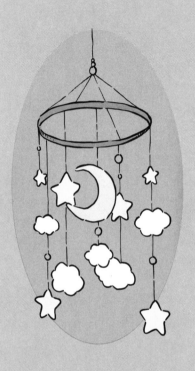

the soothing sage

Sometimes your baby is just an asshole for no reason at all.

We all have our moods. You know the ones you don't even know you're in until you've crossed a line by either saying something you instantly regret or pitching a cell phone out a second-story window? Unfortunately, the ways you level yourself out aren't applicable here: You cannot take a newborn to your favorite spa; you cannot plop them in a hot tub or pour them a cocktail. You can't tell them to take a walk or work on their intentional breathing. Retail therapy is a no-go. They don't care about new clothes or new toys or new anything, for that matter, since they're pretty new themselves. Since you're the one they count on for everything, it's your job to calm them by being all of these things. You're the dirty martini, the meditation app, the yoga instructor—the soothing sage—there to take them down from a ten.

Babies are mini-humans, but human nonetheless. This is good news. Humans, most of them, can be reasoned with regardless of size.

Start by considering their environment. Your anxiety level is not going to drop if you walk into a rocking nightclub or a rowdy sports bar, right? In your baby's difficult moments, treat your home the way a masseuse treats their parlor. No cell phones: Turn those ringers off. When you're trying to calm your baby down, the last thing you need is Beethoven's Fifth alerting you to a call from your boss. Dim the lights, mute the television, and whisk her away from anyone and anything high energy. His fight-or-flight instinct is on high alert, and any further stimulation will exacerbate the problem.

There are three golden rules when getting an irrational baby or toddler to disengage from their tantrum. 1) Distract; 2) Distract; 3) Distract. (Please feel free to take notes.) Babies have the attention span of a freaking goldfish. Nine times out of ten, if you hold up their favorite toy or treat and change the tone of your voice, they'll forget all about whatever was ailing them.

If you are going to present your baby with toys and treats to give him something else to focus on, it's important that you reveal only one talisman at a time, not a bunch of them at once. Consider how adults meditate: by focusing on a single thing, whether that's a mantra or each breath; most of us cannot effectively shut down our cognition and focus on *nothing at all*. Alternatively, we can't relax while attempting to sort out multiple things. We therefore focus on one thing and one thing only, and we make sure that thing feels relaxing or makes us content. Mimic this experience for your baby by presenting one toy at a time, until they select something that'll bring about peace and quiet.

In addition to distracting your little one, there's much more you can do to help them find bliss. The positions, holds, and massages to follow will distract and soothe the beast within.

swaddling for serenity

When you're expecting your first, everyone waxes on and on about the almighty swaddle. You'll probably get eight hundred at your shower. And if you take any don't-break-the-baby classes, they'll likely throw in a complimentary swaddle that will sit in your trunk for two years. Every mom you know will swear you'll use them as blankets, spit-up rags, car seat shields, nursing covers, emergency diapers—no judgment—and they're right.

Most babies love to be swaddled. Once you see your baby lying peacefully, bundled in a blanket more securely than any burrito you've ever had the pleasure of eating, you will have only one thing on your mind, and it ain't the burrito: "I want someone to swaddle me."

(As consenting adults with a blanket lying around the house, we highly suggest giving an adult swaddle a try. It's a warm and cozy thing to do when you're exhausted and delirious and not feeling any kind of sexy—so basically anytime within the first six months of parenthood. Alas, the following instructions are meant not for you—wink, wink—but for your security-seeking baby.)

Babies love being swaddled because it reminds them of being in the womb. This compact, cuddly position is safe and familiar, and it can be sleep-essential when they're newborns, as it helps moderate their startle (Moro) reflex, which rudely wakes them from their slumber. That said, not all babies appreciate being wrapped like a spicy salmon roll, and that's okay.

As far as fabric, we appreciate muslin for being a light material that prevents overheating. We also like a cotton blend with a bit of stretch to make it easier to get a snug fit. To keep things real, we mostly used the idiot-proof versions that you just zip, Velcro, or snap, but we still old-school swaddled on occasion. Why? Because we legitimately had eight hundred of them. Here's our tried-and-true technique for a snuggly tot:

1. Lay baby's blanket on a flat surface with the corners aimed north, south, east, and west, like a diamond.
2. Fold the top corner of the blanket over toward the center. Any former or current paper-airplane builders out there should be familiar with this move.
3. Lay your baby faceup on the blanket. They should

be centered left to right with their back on top of the fold you just made. Their head should poke above the folded edge of the blanket.

4. Lay baby's left arm straight down along their side and fold the right corner of the blanket across to secure their arm in place. Tuck the corner under the baby's back just below their right armpit.

5. Bring the bottom of the blanket up to this same spot, covering the baby's feet, and tuck it under.

6. Now wrap the left corner of the blanket over their right arm and body and tuck it into the blanket under their left side.

7. Snuggle your immobilized, contented little bean like you will never get to snuggle them again. Once they can roll over or get their arms out on their own, this game is over—this one is exclusively for newbies.

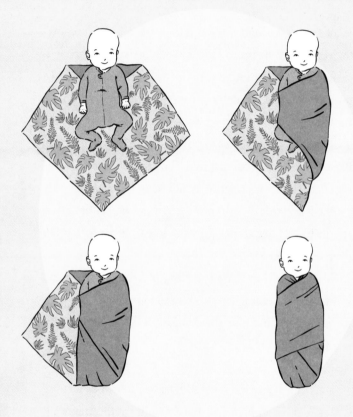

ganesha's trunk

Walt Disney's *Dumbo*, the original, left a big impression on Tony when he was a kid. When our daughter arrived, seeing her cry reminded him of the sentimental flick. In the movie, Dumbo's mother drops her trunk down through the bars of the train car where she's been jailed and soothes a sad baby Dumbo by slowly rocking him back and forth like a pendulum. This inspired Tony to try a similar technique. Like the little elephant, our daughter was instantly soothed, and this became our go-to move for her first year. It still makes her smile from ear to ear as we swing her from knee to knee.

Next time your babe is feeling frenzied, distract and soothe with this smooth swaying motion. The back-and-forth of the swing plus the comfort of being close to you equals one happy baby.

1. Create a base for yourself by spreading your feet shoulder-width apart. Bend slightly at the knee and bend forward even more slightly at the waist.

2. Create a swing out of your arms by locking your

wrists against baby's hips and firmly gripping her thighs.

3. Slowly, safely, swing your baby from side to side, tilting her backward enough to guarantee she stays secure in your arms.

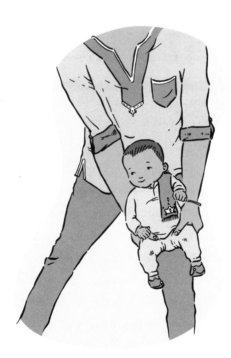

hamilton's hold

Thirty-six million viewers and counting don't lie: This two-handed grip, which was made YouTube famous by Dr. Robert Hamilton of Santa Monica, is the crème de la crème. Like so many others, we found it extremely effective at getting our girl from mad to mild.

We've been lucky enough to consult with Dr. Hamilton on his go-to move. He explained that it is so effective because you're essentially swaddling your baby with your hands, creating a feeling of security. Also, babies don't like to be completely flat; by keeping them upright, you're keeping them in their preferred position. And by rocking them, you're signaling their parasympathetic nervous system—the opposite of fight or flight. Finally, you're distracting them with the soothing movements. They forget about what's ailing them because they are now thinking, "Hey, what's happening?" It's this combination of feeling and reflex that works on fussiness.

It's important to pay attention to the angle of your baby's body, as the good doctor points out. Keeping them tilted forty-five degrees forward will assure that they remain under your loving but firm control. As baby gets larger and begins to develop more strength and more ability to flail out of your arms, the difficulty level for this hold goes up and the efficacy goes down. This occurs at a different rate for all babies, but Dr. Hamilton finds it works extremely well for the first two to three months. You'll know when it's time to move on.

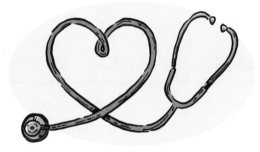

1. Pick up your baby, folding their left and right arms together across their chest.

2. Hold their arms in place with the bottom half of your palm while using the upper part of your hand, the scoop between your thumb and forefinger, to secure the baby's chin, curling your fingers beneath to stabilize and support baby's head and neck.

3. Cup your other hand around the baby's diaper and under their bottom, keeping them leaning forward at a forty-five-degree angle.

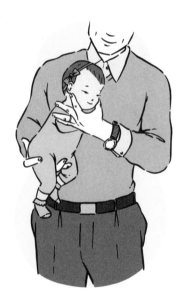

4. Softly bounce the baby: Jiggle just their bottom, or stir them around in circles like a witch stirring a potion in her cauldron, the end result of which is a spell cast over their gloom.

happy cow

The Happy Cow is so named because its motion is a lot like milking one. In fact, we've seen similar moves referred to as Indian Milking Massage and Swedish Milking Massage, but our baby loves cows (or at least mooing like one), so we're taking our inspiration from her.

You may be thinking that your squirmy baby, with the attention span of a grapefruit, won't stay still long enough to have a diaper changed, let alone indulge in a head-to-toe rubdown. That's what we thought, too, but this was not the case. Even the most high-voltage adults can enjoy a short spa session, and babies are no different. We were surprised by how easily our wiggly, willful, and independent "I-do-it" daughter took to this technique.

The Happy Cow loosens up the hardworking muscles in baby's arms and legs. Babies are constantly using new muscles as their skills extend from tummy time to terrorizing your shelves. They get aches and knots just like the rest of us! We give our girl this massage post bath, right before her longest sleep, and we believe it's the perfect way to end her day.

We suggest using a food-based oil or infant-friendly lotion (always dye-free and perfume-free).

1. Warm the oil or lotion in your hands while asking your baby permission to start the massage.

2. Hold her ankle in your left hand to support her leg. Using your right hand, cup her leg at the top of the thigh. Glide down making long, easy strokes down both sides of her leg from upper thigh to ankle, as if you're milking a cow.

3. When you reach her ankle, use your thumbs to lightly massage the arch of her foot. Pressure should be firm but gentle.

4. Repeat these strokes several times before moving on to the other leg.

5. Move your attention to the baby's arm from her armpit to wrist. If she's making a fist, use delicate strokes to get her to relax and open her hand.

6. Run your thumb across her palms, and give each finger a little love, too.

7. Repeat on the other arm.

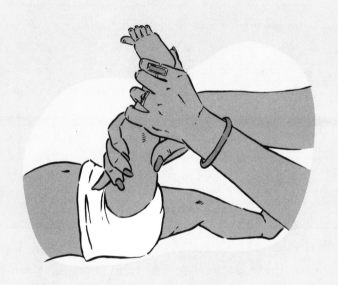

little spoon

You know how secure and comforted it makes you feel when you're lying in bed and your better half snuggles up to your back? Tony never gets that feeling because Allie doesn't like to be touched while she sleeps. Allie claims spooning is controversial, and her proof is an article she once read that listed twenty-four reasons why people hate spooning. Tony thinks she's making that up and that it is a fantastic feeling everyone enjoys but her. Allie argues that spooning, at best, leads to forking, and if it doesn't, it's just a waste of time that could be better spent sleeping.

Anyway, despite all the controversy among adults, babies love to be the little spoon. Being on their side makes them feel secure, as it reminds them of the feeding position, and the comfort of your warmth and heartbeat remind them of their time in the womb. All this plus the added bonus of facing out so they are able to take in the exciting world around them. It is the ultimate cuddle.

Next time your babe is fussing, try putting them in this position, either swaddled or not, while walking and lightly bouncing. The motion will further remind them of being inside Mom's belly.

1. Cradle your baby in your arms, facing away from you, using your upper arm and elbow to securely support the head and neck. Use your opposite hand to stabilize their chest and chin as needed.
2. Bring baby to your body, lovingly securing her back against your belly or chest.
3. Bounce, sway, or just lie there and watch the game.

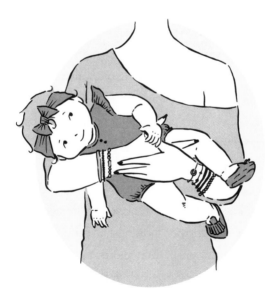

teething sucks

Seeing those adorable pearly whites peeking through is thrilling and picture-worthy every millimeter along the way for new parents. For our babies, not so much. We can't put a cute spin on this one. Teething sucks. It just does. It wakes them up, makes them fussy and mad, and kills everyone's good time. We can't imagine how excruciating it must be to have a tooth cutting its way through our gums. Second worst to experiencing it is standing by, wishing you could do something, anything, to ease their pain. Frozen washcloths, cold teething rings, and other objects to chew on offer only temporary help.

But there is another way. According to Dr. Amy Albright, DACM, there are a number of pressure points in the body for a baby experiencing tooth terrors. The most prominent is called "union valley." It exists in the dip between your thumb and forefinger, at the top of the muscle in the middle of the second metacarpal bone. It is quite sensitive. We recommend locating it on yourself first (you'll know it when you push on it) and using extra care when lightly applying pressure to your baby's hand. Keep in mind that babies experience pressure more acutely than we do. If they are at all uncomfortable, which they'll tell you by communicating nonverbally, stop.

1. With extremely light pressure, use your thumb to press on your baby's union valley.
2. Hold this pressure for ten to thirty seconds.
3. Release and repeat on your baby's other hand.
4. Alternate hands for a total of three to five minutes or until the baby is over it. This can be done up to six times daily as long as the area doesn't become tender for the baby.

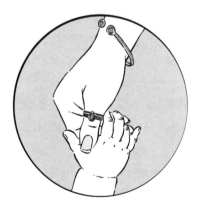

point a to point b

People kept telling us we were brave to take our baby on a flight, but we just wanted to get the hell out of town. And we did, early and often. As soon as the doctor gave us the okay to travel, we were wheels up. Puerto Vallarta, Hood River, Scottsdale, Vegas, Cape Cod, all before she reached her tenth month on the outside. Ambitious? Sure. We worried, just like every parent, that our frequent flier would be *that* kid throwing a fit on the plane and ruining the experience for everyone. But it doesn't take courage to travel with a young baby; it just takes some understanding of common potential irritants, like boredom and pressure changes. Help your baby avoid and resolve discomfort due to changes in cabin pressure, which can cause pain in their tiny ears.

Massage these points during takeoff and landing, before the pressure has a chance to build up:

1. Tucked just behind the earlobe where the jaw meets the skull, you will find a depression that your fingertip naturally falls into. Gently press and rub

here for fifteen seconds, then release for five
seconds. Repeat three times.

2. Immediately in front of the tragus, the flap of
   cartilage in front of the ear where some might have
   a piercing, there is a space that, again, your fingertip
   naturally falls into. Softly press and hold for fifteen
   seconds, then release for five seconds. Repeat
   three times.

3. Repeat steps one and two on both ears as needed
   (or as long as your baby will allow).

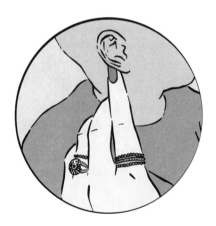

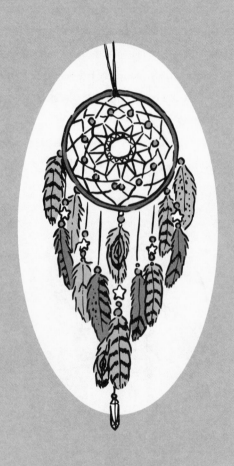

dreamy diviner

People say being a parent is exhausting, and it is. Not parenting, mind you. Being a parent. What's the difference? Feeding your baby, changing your baby, rocking your baby, and helping your baby deal with all the little issues we've already addressed, that's parenting. And yes, it's all work. And some days, that work can be tiring, especially if you are juggling it with all the other responsibilities you had before the All-Consuming One showed up. However, none of it is truly grueling on the gray matter if you've got gas in the tank. In short, *being a parent* (the noun) expresses something that *parenting* (from the verb) does not—namely, that you're doing all of the parenting stuff, which you would otherwise truly enjoy, while not having slept for days, weeks, or even months.

There is no magic book or swaddle that will make your child embrace the concept of uninterrupted sleep. There will be sleepless nights for all. Oh, we've all heard the stories of the chosen ones blessed with a unicorn child who sleeps from 7:00 p.m. to 7:00 a.m. within mere weeks of being born. "It's nothing we did. She just sleeps. She just loves to sleep. Sleep, sleep, sleep!" Fuck off. Skip ahead. This chapter is not for you.

For everyone else, all you normal people out there, we relate. For the first five or so months, we were sleepwalking clichés. Diaper cream on the toothbrush? Check! Sobbing at 2:00 a.m. over spilled breast milk? Check! Sobbing for absolutely no reason at all? CHECK! Please take heart, though. Before you shove a pillow over your face to muffle your scream-cries so you don't wake the baby, who finally decided to sleep twenty minutes before you have to leave for an appointment (check!), know that you are not without recourse. There are things you can do to increase the odds that they will require less persuasion to fall asleep in the first place, and, if all goes according to plan (ha!), sleep even longer once they do go down.

"Sleep when the baby sleeps." These words kept us up at night when we could have been sleeping. Everyone will advise you in the early months of parenthood to abandon your laundry list of things to do and drift off. Everyone, from strangers on the street to the pizza delivery guy. It's like one person tried it and the whole world jumped on the bandwagon, whether they believed it to be possible or not. The concept makes sense: Babies cannot conform to your schedule, and you cannot bribe them into submission. If you can't beat them, join them, right? Well, for us, this was wrong. But not because we wanted it to be! Our anxieties about all the other things (e.g., Did we walk the dog? Do we have groceries for dinner? Did I brush my teeth today?) turned on the second our little lady turned off. If you were able to actually sleep when your baby slept, we salute you.

Having exhausted this possibility, we resigned ourselves to working with her to get her to sleep through the night as quickly as possible. We relied on sources of knowledge and skill outside the realm of our local barista or the woman next door whose last baby was born before *The Wizard of Oz*. We turned instead to the worlds of sensory stimulation and energy work—both of which have relaxed us at various points—and found that they held exactly the secrets we needed in order to routinely knock her sweet tush out.

We were incredibly lucky to consult with the king of good energy, Dr. John Amaral. For those not in the know, Dr. Amaral, a chiropractor, energy healer, and educator, works with celebrities, pro athletes, and high-powered CEOs to elevate their energy so they feel and perform their best. What many of his fans and clients don't know is that John and his wife, Christina, also a chiropractor and energy and body healer, have helped hundreds of babies, too! Midwives, doulas, lactation consultants, family physicians, and pediatricians often refer their young patients who are having difficulty sleeping to Dr. and Dr. Amaral.

We were incredibly lucky to meet Dr. John through a friend when Kingsley was only a few months old. Our baby was pretty fussy from the start and wasn't sleeping as well as her same-age friends. As soon as John met her, he shocked us by intuiting that she'd gotten stuck in the birth canal on her way out. He explained that she, too, had experienced trauma during the birth (something we hadn't even considered) and was holding on to that tension in her little neck. After a few minutes of energy work, our daughter exploded into her diaper, which he had warned us would happen. It was like a light had been switched on: Our baby was suddenly more relaxed in general, went to sleep more easily, and stayed asleep longer. In short: All hail Dr. Amaral!

These are the techniques he recommends to parents to help their infant calm down by preparing their body for sleep. Hopefully they allow a weary parent to drift off to a deep dreamy sleep as well. The moves work by increasing the tone of your vagus nerve (vagal tone), which activates the parasympathetic nervous system, often referred to as the "rest and digest" system. Meaning your body can come down faster after stress.

> The vagus nerve is the longest in your body, connecting your brain to many vital organs, including your gut, heart, and lungs. The word *vagus* means "wanderer" in Latin, representing how the nerve wanders throughout the body.

The most important factor in getting your baby to wind down is breathing, relaxing, and tuning in to your own body first, which then helps you to better tune in to your baby's energy and rhythm. You will transfer and translate your emotional state through the way you breathe and touch your baby, and through the transfer of your overall energy, which will transform your baby in the process. Check in with yourself first, then proceed to your baby.

om sweet om

Visualize, if you will, a solitary monk sitting cross-legged with his eyes closed, humming his way to nirvana. It is no doubt to us that this actually *works*. I mean, when was the last time you were flipped off by a monk? Yeah, us neither. This isn't because they don't experience the same spectrum of emotions as the rest of us. It's because they Om their way through that shit. And you can, too.

Dr. Amaral taught us that humming or OM'ing increases your vagus tone and thereby calms you down. The calmer you are, the more you can tune in to your baby. Your humming or OM'ing will also create a physical vibration in your baby's body, and the more "coherent" (at ease and in flow) you are, the more that calming murmur will relax her, letting her slip into sleep.

1. Hold your baby against your chest, facing you.
2. Begin to take deep, long, slow breaths into your belly. This is called diaphragmatic breathing, and it is a proven way to relax your nervous system.

3. On the exhale, begin to hum. Hum an "OM" sound, or a tune, or any vibration in the back of your throat that feels good.

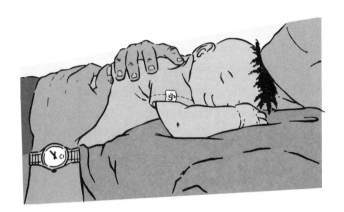

blossoming lotus

The lotus flower is considered the most spiritually in tune of blossoms because of its phenomenal life cycle. Its roots are planted in mud, and every night it submerges into the muck. At daylight, it reemerges and seemingly miraculously reblooms, with no evidence of its murky evening. We see ourselves—or all parents, for that matter—in the lotus flower. No matter what shit, literal or otherwise, we were covered in the night before, we emerge the next morning ready to start anew.

The Blossoming Lotus works by stimulating the vagus nerve, which directly serves the heart and gut and passes through the diaphragm. Delicately soothing these three areas can help to regulate the autonomic nervous system, inducing calm and rest.

1. Bring the fingertips and thumb of one hand together loosely to form a relaxed point.
2. With your baby on her back, place this point gently on her chest and spread your fingers apart very slowly and delicately, envisioning a lotus flower

blossoming open as you do so. Repeat this three times.

3. Now move your fingertips to her solar plexus (middle of body at diaphragm) and repeat three times.

4. Then, move your fingertips to her belly and once again repeat three times.

5. After you have bloomed the lotus in each of these areas, very softly draw your fingertips up from her belly in a line across her solar plexus and back up to her heart. You can repeat this sequence as many times as you'd like.

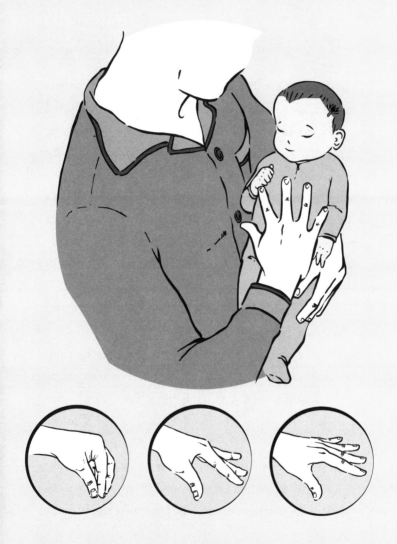

sleepy swirls

Your baby takes their cues from you. They look to you to learn everything from expressions, to funny animal noises, to more complex things like language and swiping through pictures on your phone. They also look to you for mood and for how they should be feeling in a given moment. If you feel scared, they will feel that, too. That's right, they will learn to emulate your energy. If you want to have a relaxed baby, one who can be tuned to be ready for sleep, you yourself must first relax and feel ready for sleep as well.

Before approaching your baby, breathe deeply and unwind your own mind and body. Once you've achieved calm, share this emotional state with your baby by daintily swirling your fingers across their back while imagining a soothing energy flowing from you through your baby's entire body, relaxing and drifting them into a deep sleep.

The nerves that supply the adrenal glands exit the spine between the tenth thoracic and the first lumbar vertebrae, which is right around the bottom of the rib cage.

This is where you want to focus. Think of these nerves as the receptors you need to plug into in order to transmit your emotional state.

1. Hold your baby against your chest, facing you.
2. Swirl your fingertips over your baby's mid and lower back on either side of the spine in slow, rhythmic spirals.

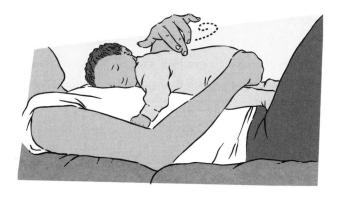

twilight tickles

You know in a horror movie when the villain is *finally* down and out and our heroes are sharing a victory hug, relieved that the danger is over and they can get on with their lives? What happens? The bad guy springs awake for one last scare before being put away for good. Every. Time. We're convinced this genre cliché was originally thought up by a parent who had trouble putting their kid to sleep. We know you've been there. Your baby, lulled lovingly in your arms, is displaying all of the visible and audible signs of being in a deep, deep sleep. Mouth slightly ajar. Delicious snores. Limp as a string of angel hair. But the moment after you lay them down and start army crawling away, that's when they grab your ankle, dragging you back to the battlefield of bedtime.

These tickles are a simple way to manipulate your boo's brain chemistry so they sink right back into slumber. The chemical in play is oxytocin, otherwise known as the love hormone. Oxytocin is released when the sensory nerves are activated through positive, warm, skin-to-skin interactions. This light tickle of a touch also stimulates the release of dopamine in the brain, an important neurotransmitter. The moment to practice this move is when baby is in that fragile fleeting state teetering between awake and asleep. Works every time.

1. Lightly and slowly brush your fingertips down your baby's forehead, nose, and the sides of her cheeks while shushing quietly.
2. Change up your pattern but stay consistent in the barely there pressure of your touch.
3. Pay close attention to her reaction. You might see her give the slightest, sweetest smile before drifting off to sleep.

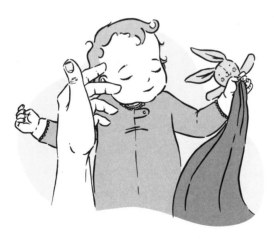

third eye touch

You're lying in bed. Your eyes are closed. You're exhausted and want nothing more than to go to sleep. The problem is, your mind is racing and you don't know why. You haven't had caffeine since breakfast. You got paid today, and the check was bigger than expected. On top of all that positivity, you were able to dim the lights an hour before bedtime, shut off your television and phone, and spend the last hour reading a book on how to achieve better sleep. But for some reason, the sheep you're counting are zombie sheep, armed to the teeth, and they are hunting you.

In moments like this, it's the hands of others that provide the most comfort. Touch is a powerful sedative, especially when it's sweet, slow, and applied to the right places—no, not *there*. We're talking about the face. When energy gets congested in the head, it can cause the restlessness we've just described. This is especially true for babies. The good news is, babies' energy is more malleable than yours, and they are extremely sensitive to touch. Once you learn to clear their blockages, relief is just seconds away.

1. Placing your forefinger just above the center of the eyebrows, begin feather-light downward strokes to the bridge of the nose. Match the rate of the stroke with the state of baby's wakefulness: Begin slow . . . and then go even slower as the baby nears sleep. Make sure you always move your finger downward, as this is the direction we want the energy to move.

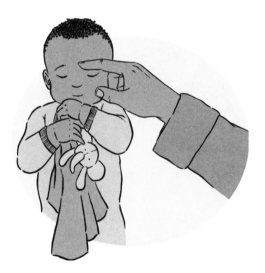

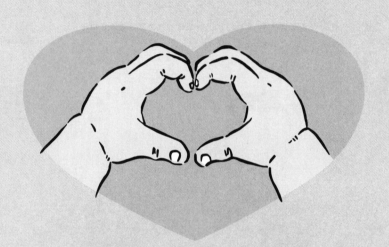

sensory sensei

In today's world, many of us think of mind and body as separate entities. This is a misunderstanding. There is no mind apart from the body, just as there is no body apart from the mind. There is only the whole of the mindbody, and how that single entity learns and develops through the seven senses.

That's right, we said *seven* senses. Many of you, like us, learned about the five external senses early on: sight, sound, taste, smell, and touch. There are two internal sensory systems, as well: the proprioceptive and the vestibular. Wait, the what and the WHAT?

The vestibular system is your sense of balance and motion. The fluid in your inner ear sends signals so you can sense the overall position and rate of motion of your body. It tells you when you're moving, how fast, and in what direction. It also allows you to coordinate between your left and right sides, which includes head and eye movement.

The proprioceptive system is your sense of position. It tells you where your body is in relation to other objects. When your sense of balance and motion tells you you're running at full speed, your sense of position keeps you from running face-first into a brick wall. It also tracks what your body parts are up to and determines how much force is required to do tasks, like picking up a ball or throwing it through a hoop.

We spend a lot of time worrying about what to do for our baby when they're uncomfortable or in a bad mood, but what do we do with them when they're in a good mood (aside from taking lots of pictures)? We play with them, of course! Play is critical to helping your baby develop a healthy and happy mindbody. But how do infants play? It's not like they can do, well, anything.

Giving the seven senses a solid workout not only encourages learning and physical growth, it helps with all the other issues we've covered: constipation, mood, lack of sleep, and irregular sleep patterns. We found that this was especially true when it came to getting z's. Baby brains are always churning and learning, reaching and growing, so the more you give each of their senses to process while their eyes are open, the easier their eyes will close and the longer they will stay that way.

If you want your baby to sleep when you want them to sleep, wake them up—not from actual sleep, but to the world. And you do that by stimulating the shit out of them. Really—some new babies will actually soil their diaper in response to playtime. Becoming a sensory sensei is not just a great way to maximize the enjoyment and bonding with your new baby, but a necessary part of any comprehensive campaign to keep your little one on an ideal schedule.

Read on to learn how to increase melatonin (the sleep hormone), decrease cortisol (the stress hormone), and destroy any other barrier to your babe's downtime.

start toying with them

Give Them Space

The silver, crinkly blankets commonly found in emergency kits are also known as space blankets. These lightweight throws are not only real-world lifesavers, they're also incredibly exciting to infants. For one, they're reflective, sparkly, and fun to look at (stimulating their sense of sight). Two, the loud crunch sound draws your baby's attention like no other toy can (sound). They love pinching, squishing, and—as they get older—playing peek-a-boo with it. For pre-crawlers, lay them on top of the blanket (on their back or for tummy time) listening to the sounds they make with every wiggle.

Important note: These blankets are not toys, nor are they to be used as actual blankets. They require your full supervision at all times.

Spilled Silk

At first, we didn't understand why every playgroup we attended had rainbow-colored silky squares, but soon we were converts. Babies love gathering and discovering these soft-to-the-touch (and apparently quite tasty) silks. Unlike other toys, they are easy to grab hold of and won't roll away. For a multisensory activity at any age, take the silk and drape it delicately over your baby from head to toe. He'll love the tickly sensation (touch). Throw the silks into the air and entertain him with the flying colors (sight).

All Wound Up

Wind-up toys make a big impression. When babes see and hear those brightly colored animals or bugs zipping across the room, they get so jazzed. This activity is not

only invigorating for sight and sound; it encourages movement since your babe will track them as they scoot by, and
eventually they'll be motivated to roll over and grab those
little suckers as they go.

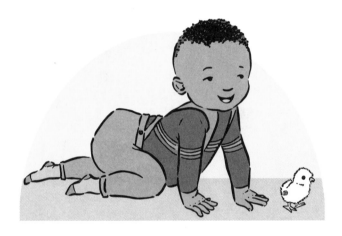

play with their food

As soon as they're able, anything your baby can get their hands on they will put in their mouth. One of our constant battles as a parent is to make sure everything that touches their tongue is clean and safe. But this oral exploration stage is key to their development, so why should we lean away from this natural instinct when we can lean in? Playtime with food plays a huge part in developing their senses of sight and touch in addition to taste and smell, and Lisa Eberly Mastela—registered dietician, nutritionist, and mother of two—recommends bringing food into playtime and play into mealtime. For instance, go ahead and give them a spoon and a bowl of yogurt early on instead of spoon-feeding them. Will this result in a mess? You betcha. It will also give them space to explore and practice the external senses we've already mentioned, while simultaneously engaging the internal senses of balance, motion, and position. Additionally, getting their hands a little messy allows them to investigate new textures and flavors in a fun and engaging way. Even better, this makes them more likely to be willing to try unfamiliar and unexpected foods.

Try to think of the inevitable cleanup as an investment in your and your little one's future confidence and ability to self-service. That's right! You can chisel away at that oatmeal ingrained on your hardwoods with an eye toward your own self-care. As parents we often sacrifice eating our own meals (taking turns, or shoveling food down at the speed of light) while assisting our kids. Letting them make messes now will likely lead to them eating expertly from a spoon *on their own* much faster than peers who were spoon-fed, freeing you up to enjoy your own dinner while it's still hot.

PRO-TIP: Mastela says that it can take up to fifteen tries before baby will learn to like a new food or flavor. At first (and maybe even at the tenth attempt), they may ignore it, purse their lips, or throw away a bite before they will risk putting it in their mouth, but rejection doesn't necessarily mean that they don't like it; it usually means they simply aren't ready. Offering a variety of different tastes and textures will diversify their palate over the long term, so stay persistent and mix it up by introducing a new flavor every few days: Try Indian spices, then

Mexican, or Italian, and so on. Give leftovers as snacks to help them "meet" these fresh flavors again and again until they're ready to accept and enjoy!

Noodle Pool

This one is for the braver of parents because, well, pasta gets everywhere—and we mean *everywhere*. But anything for the kids, right? *Right?*

Cook up at least two adult servings of spaghetti, letting them boil a few minutes longer for extra squishiness. Once they are completely cooled down, they're ready to go. The great thing about pasta play is that you don't have to worry about it going in their mouth (taste!), as almost all things do, since it's edible. We put our baby in a seat in the bathtub and let her go to town. However, some (cooler) parents we know have filled an entire plastic pool for a full-on spaghetti immersion.

Stacking Sweets

Two things all babies love to do are stack and squish. This activity helps develop eye-hand coordination while indulging their young taste buds with a sweet treat.

With your baby in his high chair, have him build, arrange, smash, and explore a variety of fruit. Cut large pieces from fruits such as cantaloupe, honeydew, and watermelon into cubes and other fun shapes too big to fit into his mouth.

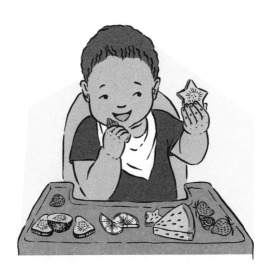

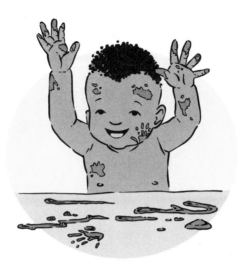

Le Petit Artiste

Immediately after placing anything pureed in front of your new eater, they poke their little fingers in and inspect what is soon to be a big mess. If your goal is to get them to actually consume the stuff, it doesn't allow for too much play, so we like the idea of a time apart from meals when you can allow their curiosity to run wild without worrying about whether they're getting enough calories. We give our girl a few dollops of colorful purees to finger paint as she pleases—on the tray of her high chair, on her body, across a canvas, whatever. If you're feeling extra, you can whip up your own edible paints by blending up purple potato, yams, carrots, peas, and so on. But no judgment whatsoever if you purchase premade pouches and call it a day. (This is our preferred route, truth be told.)

let there be beats!

Music can do so much more than soothe the savage beast. For babes it also serves as an early conduit for learning to recognize patterns. As humans, that ability is what sets us and our little monkeys apart from all the other animals in the world.

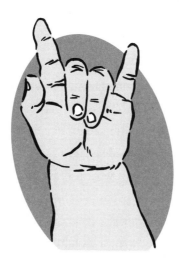

For years, parents living in Southern California have known all about the BeatBuds, musical partners who create catchy tunes aimed to educate and entertain infants and children of all ages. The wildly popular band is beloved by little ones—some might say obsessively. They're in high demand for birthday parties, group classes, and even concerts at some of L.A.'s most notorious (grown-up) venues.

Before we were parents, we thought we could coax our future kid into loving our favorite bands. We weren't going to be those parents listening to "The Wheels on the Bus" over and over and over again. So naïve were we. Once our baby was old enough to sit up, she was taking group music classes with the BeatBuds and absolutely thriving because of them. Her motor skills improved. She lit up for certain songs. She could play instruments properly. There was something about that music that not only got her jamming but made her grow.

We wanted to know what it is about children's music that makes the littles so damn happy, and more than that, what about music class is so essential to their growth and development, so we went right to the source. We spoke to the BeatBuds about song selection for infants and toddlers, how it is designed, and why it seems to have such a hold on little minds and ears. You'll soon learn, if you haven't already, that most babies will have no interest in what's on your playlist. They will, however, happily listen to "The Wheels on the Bus" over and over and over and over and over and over and over, before crying with displeasure when you finally reach your limit.

The repetitious nature of "family music" (as the Beat-Buds like to call it) makes a ton of sense, though. The simpler the pattern and the more it repeats, the easier it is for them to grasp and enjoy. Likewise, they're comprised of short one- and two-syllable words about simple objects and simple actions. The more we learned about the design behind family music, the more we came to enjoy listening to it. Recognizing the patterns behind those artistic choices actually gave us a feeling of learning, too—nope, that's a lie. We still want to bang our heads into a wall whenever "The Wheels on the . . ."—you know.

I bet you never considered that plastic baby rattle a musical instrument, but that's exactly what it is, and the sooner your baby learns to shake it in time with the beat, the sooner they'll be onstage at Carnegie Hall or the Whisky a Go Go. Whenever your baby can grasp your pinky finger, they can also grasp a tambourine or an egg shaker. And once they learn to sit up, they can hold a stick and beat it against a drum.

Instrument play is a way to engage children through sight, touch, and sound. At their classes, the BeatBuds distribute one simple percussion instrument at a time to stimulate engagement. Every household should keep a few of these favorites around the house for baby to play with while their favorite tunes are blasting through the speakers.

Instruments of Change

Egg shaker
Tambourine
Maracas
Bongo drum
Xylophone
Handbells

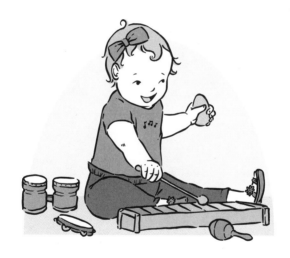

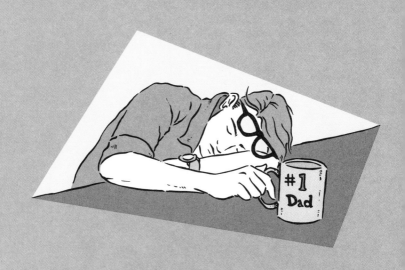

the achy creator

Decades of commitment to physical fitness did nothing to prepare us for the first year of parenthood. Tony previously spent seven days a week surfing, getting pummeled by the Pacific Ocean and coming out of the water feeling on top of the world. Likewise, Allie spent every day writing in a sports club so on her writing breaks she could run, lift, maybe take a Pilates class. We tested and challenged our bodies, and our bodies met those challenges daily. Before we got pregnant, we were strong, pain free, energy rich, and reasonably sexy.

Nine months of pregnancy plus twelve months of child-rearing have not only erased our former aesthetic, which we both agree it would be nice to have back, but, more significantly, jettisoned any trace of our former strength and energy. Priorities inevitably shift. Sex has not gone completely out the window, but the window is open and sex is teetering on the sill, staring down at a four-story drop with its life passing before its eyes. We haven't lost interest in each other, and we do still enjoy sex when it occurs. But who has the time or energy when we are so far behind on the last season of *The Bachelor*? Allie could put on the sexiest lingerie in the world and saunter into the bedroom with a glass of top-shelf scotch over a single cube of ice and declare, "I'll do anything," and Tony would roll over onto his stomach, motion to his shoulder, and say, "I've got a knot right here."

Pregnancy and parenting are going to kick your ass time and again. The good news is that you will enjoy every minute of it. Your baby will fill you with love and joy in a way you never imagined possible, while simultaneously decimating your ability to stand up without grunting and groaning. Strains, knots, twists, pulls, and tears are no longer a risk of ambitious promiscuity or feats of athleticism; they are the result of tending to our ever-growing, ever-squirmier dependent. All of the positions you've read about so far, along with any other you might find yourself in, will challenge your load-bearing undercarriage in ways a kettlebell, treadmill, or fuzzy handcuffs never did. You will find yourself in asymmetrical postures, bent forward or leaning to one side, more often than not, inevitably throwing off your body's natural balance.

Being a parent means bearing five to fifty pounds of extra weight on one side—and probably one side only, as research shows that we tend to always carry a baby the same way, because we are more dexterous with one hand, which we want to leave free. Additionally, babies prefer—nay, demand—routine. They will grow fond of whatever they're accustomed to. If you start out carrying on your right side, leaving your left hand free for the phone, coffee mug, or keyboard, just try switching your three-month-old to the left side. It's not happening. If they're used to being on the right, the right is where they want to be, and it has absolutely nothing to do with political affiliation.

Imagine going to the gym and only exercising your right side every day for months on end, leaving the left side to atrophy. For every action there is an equal and opposite pain in your back, your neck, your arm, and so on. You can't expect to stay balanced if you keep taking two steps forward and never two steps back.

Think of the stretches and positions we present in here as those exquisite two steps back. They will help you compensate for the lopsided strain you're putting on your body—the needed checks for those imbalances. No equipment or formal training is required, just time. How much? It depends. As in all things, when it comes to physical pain brought on by parenthood, prevention is mostly about awareness. It's important to remind yourself, "Okay, I've been nursing or massaging or scrolling Instagram for a million minutes; I have to counterbalance my neck posture for something resembling an equal amount of time." It depends on the amount of luxury you have at your disposal. Hell, yes, we just referred to time as luxury; Gucci ain't got nothing on delicious *time*. If you have three minutes to spare, good news: You can work on one targeted area. Fifteen minutes free? You can manage your entire body and upper torso. Twenty to thirty? Okay, let's not delve into the realm of fantasy here. We know your time is limited, but you must budget some of whatever you've got to take care of yourself physically in order to better take care of everyone else.

When you're on a flight, the attendants will instruct you to put on your oxygen mask before helping others do the same. This is the put-your-mask-on-before-assisting-others chapter. Refer to it frequently.

hip hiker

Carrying your kid on your hip is inevitable. You are, for the time being, a pony, and your pelvis is the saddle. As much as our bodies cry in pain, we cry happy tears for the opportunity to be our boo's personal Mister Ed. Despite the bitching, we truly do feel blessed to be her parents. We also feel warm and fuzzy to have found our chiropractor, Dr. Matt Bernstein. He educated us about hip hiking, which has helped our hips come back down to earth. Dr. B provided instruction for all the stretches in this section. Not only is he a wizard when it comes to correcting our bodies, but he's a dad (times four!), so he knows firsthand what all needs to be fixed.

In a nutshell, when we carry on our hip, we do two things to our body: We crunch down on the side we're holding, and we hike up on the other. Everyone hip hikes in order to carry their child comfortably. This posture creates a major imbalance in the body, leading to strain and tension. The quadratus lumborum muscle, or the QL, is the deepest abdominal muscle, which us non-doctors commonly refer to as our back muscle. If you're crunched and hunched to the left side, contracting tightly into the QL, you've got to counterbalance with a stretch, or you'll shorten the core muscle as it gets used to being squeezed that way. Simply stretching out in the opposite direction offers relief and increases blood flow to the compacted side.

The only way to save yourself from hip hiking is to stretch and self-correct. Opening up the QL on a regular basis will save you from so much pain—and possibly eventually having to hem just one pant leg. Just sayin'.

1. Stand with your feet shoulder-width apart.

2. Reach one arm as high up as you can.

3. Slowly allow gravity to take you over the side.

4. Keep your arm straight as you tilt as far as you can until you feel a good stretch (as with all stretches, stop if you feel any pain or discomfort).

5. Repeat with the other side.

6. Stretch each side for thirty seconds for three rounds.

frenemy stretch

You ever have one of those friends who's also sort of your nemesis? Perhaps they compliment your style to your face and then behind your back refer to your misguided fashion choice as "pulling a [your name here]"? Well, we're sorry to tell you that your baby is your frenemy. No, he's not going around talking shit about your subpar swaddling skills. What he is doing is much worse.

You're feeding your little angel. They're gazing up at you with a look that says, *You're the greatest person to ever grace this planet.* They barely *blink* because they're so mesmerized by your beauty. What you don't realize is that your sweetie is sucking the life-force straight from your spine. With every glance down, you're dipping your dome into the depths of physical hell. Your head weighs approximately ten pounds—if you've got it positioned where it's supposed to be, with your ears directly over your shoulders. When we shift from this safe place and become even the slightest amount off-kilter (i.e., looking down at your baby, checking your phone, assessing your desperate need for a pedicure), the forces of gravity cruelly add twenty to thirty pounds of pressure to our neck and spine. Yowza! Considering how often and for how long we parents are held hostage to this position, it's no wonder that our necks are constantly killing us. (You're stretching your noggin ear-to-shoulder right now, aren't you? Well, that's not going to do the trick, but we are about to tell you what does.) You need to counter all this head-hanging with a move that relieves and supports the postural muscles in your neck. Enter the frenemy stretch.

1. Take a hand towel/swaddle blanket/T-shirt/ whatever, and fold it in half by length (taco style). Roll it up.
2. Lie on the floor, and place your rolled item at the base of your skull.
3. Tilt your chin slightly upward, creating a C-shaped curve in your neck toward the floor.
4. Stay in this stretch for ten to fifteen minutes.

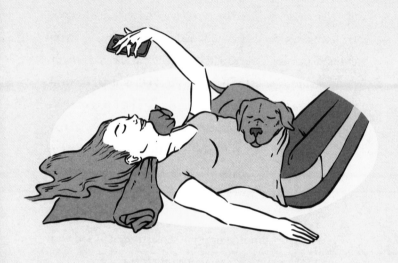

ten chin tension

This is the perfect exercise to accompany the Frenemy Stretch. Equally as important to offering relief is building up the muscles we need most, such as the ones in our neck. By going against better judgment and making as many chins as possible, you're activating the muscle group (sub-occipital muscles) at the base of your skull, which gets weak when you're looking down all the time. The irony of these muscles needing extra care due to scrolling on social media is that this move is not post-able due to your unflattering gobble-like neck. But who cares when you're #Blessed with a nicely stretched and flexed neck? Not us.

1. Sitting or standing upright, look straight ahead with your ears directly over your shoulders.
2. Pull your chin and head straight back as if you're trying to give yourself ten chins. You should feel a nice stretch at the base of your head and top of your neck.
3. Hold for five seconds, and then release to relax. Then repeat up to ten times.

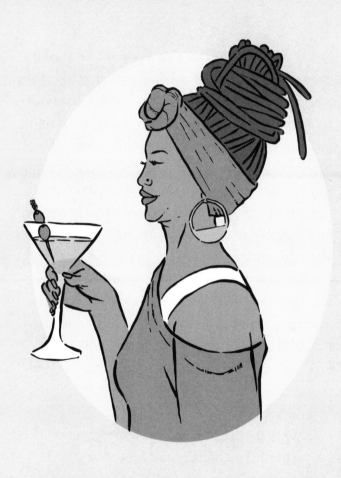

channeling chair pose

You know those inflatable air dancers that retail outlets employ to get your attention? You see them outside auto lots, marking grand openings, or in an overly festive neighbor's front yard around the holidays. No offense if you're that neighbor. We used to think they were super cheesy, but now we're just envious of them. We glare as it nimbly and smoothly whips about from head to toe, its loose, free-flowing moves inspiring sheer jealousy. Carrying young ones changes your center of gravity (hip hiking) and adds weight to your core, causing the hips and glutes to work both harder and unevenly. Things down there get tight—real tight. This awesome stretch opens up the hips by mobilizing the glutes and piriformis (the largest and most powerful muscle group in your body) while relieving lower back pain and pressure on the sciatic nerve. Doesn't that just sound fantastic? It is.

1. While standing, cross one ankle over your opposing knee, forming the shape of the number "4."

NOTE: If you need to hold on to something to complete this move, do. This is not a balancing pose. It's a stretch. Do whatever makes you feel the most stable.

2. Clasp your hands and extend them directly in front of you. This will serve as the counterbalance for the next move.

3. Sit as if you are sitting in a chair, pushing your butt back. You will feel this stretch through your hip and buttock as your center of gravity shifts into your belly. The deeper you sink into this, the more forceful the stretch will become.

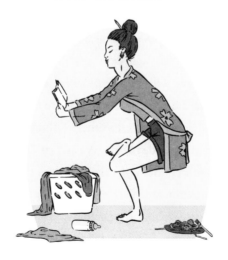

doorway to heaven

Your pecs are too tight. We don't know you, but we know this about you. If you are a human living in the age of phones and keyboards, you definitely have tight pectoral muscles. If you're reading this book, you're likely caring for babies, and, in that case, you most definitely have tight pectoral muscles. Furthermore, you don't know that this tightness is a major contributor to that persistent discomfort you feel in your shoulders and neck. You probably think this agony is due to knots and twists in your shoulders and neck. Which it could be, but guess what is aggravating your shoulder and neck, causing the knots to form? You guessed it: tight pecs.

Just like with hip hiking, when you are always stretching one side of your body, you are simultaneously shortening—tightening—the other. This applies to front and back as well as side to side. We all lean forward a disproportionate amount in this age of attention deficits, and all of this crunching means we are routinely compressing and therefore tightening our pectorals.

This door stretch is the best and simplest way to

counteract these effects, lengthening and loosening the anterior muscles in service of their neighboring joints and muscles. All you need is a doorframe (or a steady high-five from your partner) to signal a turn down Pain Free Drive.

1. Stand in an open doorway.
2. Raise both arms up at your sides, bent at ninety degrees.
3. Rest your palms on each side of the doorframe.
4. Slowly and gently lean forward. (This is where you go, "Holy shit. My pecs are crazy tight." Told you.)
5. For a deeper stretch, lean farther. This should not be painful. As with all stretches, if you feel pain, stop.
6. Hold for thirty seconds. Rest your arms. Repeat three times.

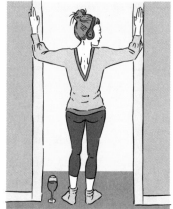

posture poses

It's an unfortunate reality of our modern lives: Whether you're a parent, a DJ, a computer nerd, or all three, most of us spend a disproportionate amount of time hunched forward. Not to worry, you are not doomed to a life of living in the shadows of a bell tower in Paris. Posture doesn't break suddenly. You won't wake up one day and suddenly find that you can no longer bend over to tie your shoes. Posture erodes slowly over time, so it follows that it will take patience and practice to restore it to the glory of your youth. The good news is that it can be done. Dr. Bernstein schooled us about our habitual discomfort, and he suggested the following two exercises to combat it.

B's Squeeze (lower rhomboids)

This is not a stretch. Repeat, this is not a stretch. Okay, that's a stretch—it is a stretch—but it's not *just* a stretch. This is a strengthening exercise meant to repair the damage done to your posture from hunching by giving your back the support and stamina it needs. The muscles we use when we hunch have all been sitting on one side of a seesaw for a very long time, waiting for someone to come play with them. The widely lauded Bruegger exercise prescribed by back doctors worldwide is just the thing they've been waiting for.

Take your time easing into this position when doing it for the first time. You are engaging elements of your body that may have been asleep for quite a while. You may feel some tingling. This is normal for nerves waking up from a long, dormant period, locked away in a cramped, dark space.

1. Stand up straight. If you find it helpful, you can stand with your back to a wall. Make sure the back of your head, your shoulders, your buttocks, and your heels are all touching the wall, without arching the small of your back. The goal here is to line up your ear directly over your shoulder. Your shoulder directly over your hip. Your hip directly with your ankle.
2. Comfortably tuck your chin straight back.
3. Press your hands together with your fingers pointing away from you.
4. Pull your shoulders down.

5. Activate your shoulder blades by opening your arms, externally rotating your arms out and back while keeping your elbows locked to your ribs.

6. Repeat ten times for three sets.

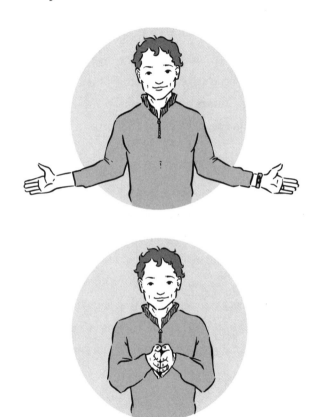

Holding, feeding, carrying, changing, dressing. Pretty much every single parental thing you do has one thing in common. (If you're thinking that's love, you're cute, but wrong.) It's rolling your shoulders inward. Curled-in shoulders are a serious source of back pain. They need to be checked before, during, and after you get wrecked. We used to do shoulder rolls thinking this would help loosen us up, but we're idiots. This is the exact wrong move. Our doctor explained that the discomfort we feel comes from our trapezius being overly activated and that shoulder rolls create even more trapezius activation. (And we were doing the whole thing without a net, too. Budumpbum.) He taught us this move designed for scapular kissing, which is a simple technique used to alleviate and reset the upper rhomboids.

Again, take your time and be intentional with these slight movements to make the most of them. You can work with what little time you have by doing them in the shower or while waiting for a bottle to warm.

1. Stand in an anatomical position, where your muscles are at their lowest tension. This means

standing straight, feet facing forward, arms at your sides with palms facing interior, and fingers pointing down. Tilt your chin slightly upward.

2. Pump your arms back, allowing the scapula "kiss," then release. Pump, pause. Pump, pause. Do this ten times.

3. Hold your arms out at ninety degrees. Pump your arms back in the same motion ten times.

4. Repeat these sets three times.

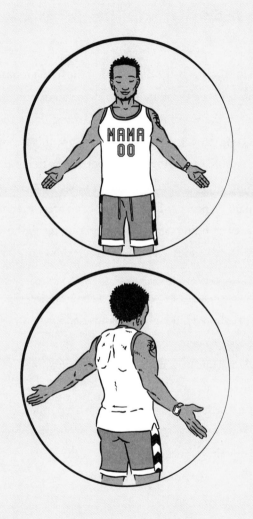

picking up the peaces

If you find yourself crawling around the living room floor, picking up toys throughout the day, you are already 70 percent of the way toward accomplishing this stretchercize. Commonly known as Cat and Cow, this move both stretches and strengthens the connective tissue around your spine. The controlled, subtle movements help with back pain, especially in the lower back area, making the process of standing back up after picking up all those toys (for the third or fourth time) easier on your entire frame.

1. Start on all fours with your weight evenly distributed among your hands and knees and your back in a neutral position.
2. Arch your back up toward the ceiling, like an angry cat.
3. Enhance this movement with a deep inhale.
4. With an exhale, tighten your abdominals and drop your chest toward the floor
5. Repeat this movement ten times.

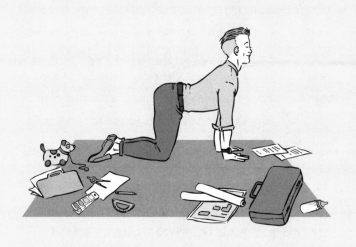

namaste right here

Bhujangasana, otherwise widely known to yogis as Cobra Pose, is the answer to the discomfort you're feeling in your back and neck. This pose increases flexibility in the spine while stretching the chest and shoulders. Those in the namaste know it can alleviate signs of stress, anxiety, and depression, too. In Sanskrit, *bhujanga* translates to "serpent" and *asana* to "pose," therefore the name. Addressing our mind, body, *and* soul in under a minute? Sign us up. You'll love this stretch so much, you're not going to want to move from it.

1. Lie flat, facing down on a comfortable surface.
2. With your legs together, your thighs and the tops of your feet should be pressed against the ground.
3. Spread your hands on the floor underneath your shoulders and hug your elbows into your rib cage.
4. Steadily straighten your arms and lift your chest toward the ceiling without pushing your ribs forward.
5. Enhance the position by using your hands to gently

press your bend farther back. Only do what is comfortable, being sure to avoid overarching your spine.

6. Stay in this position for up to twenty deep, intentional breaths.

7. Slowly release your body down to the floor in an exhale.

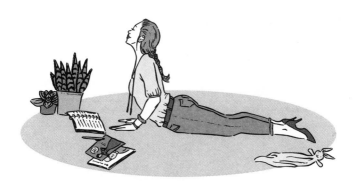

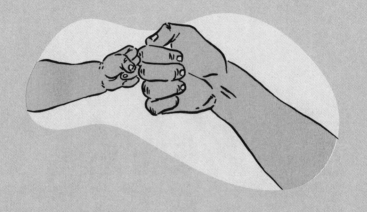

at the end of the (sometimes very long) day

Every baby leaves their little fingerprints on the world, and they all have their unique grooves. Figuring out what those are is part of the fun of being a parent. It's also a big part of the challenge. It requires the two things your baby needs from you more than anything else: time and attention. It's not a coincidence that these are the same two things that everyone and everything else in your life also requires. Whether it's your job, your partner, your favorite TV show, a hobby, or a house plant, sorting out how to divide your time and attention will *also* ironically take time and attention. Our goal is to leave you with a quick reference guide to spare as much of your time and attention while still imparting our hard-won wisdom on how to make your baby feel happy and safe.

This has been our polestar. If you ask what we want for our kid, it has nothing to do with being more advanced than her peers. Go easy on the pressure of percentiles. Don't worry about words—how many your kid can say and how quickly they begin saying them. Don't worry about steps or how soon yours takes their first one. If your kid is happy and safe, you will feel the same way, and you will have a sense of accomplishment unmatched by anything else you've ever given your time and attention to.

Here's to you and yours and all the wonderful challenges ahead. May you meet them with confidence in yourself and encouragement from all those around you! You got this! Happy parenting.

meet our experts

Much like parenthood, the Mama Sutra takes a village. We are so thankful for our tribe of genius contributors who were willing to drop their immense knowledge for the sake of our sanity . . . oh, and for the sake of our babies, too. Dr. John Amaral is a father, chiropractor, energy healer, and educator who works with successful entrepreneurs, celebrities, and pro athletes to elevate their energy so they can feel and perform their best. John, whose work is featured on Gwyneth Paltrow's *The Goop Lab* on Netflix, has worked with thousands of people from over fifty countries. His work heals physical injuries, anxiety, and depression and helps many high-achieving people maximize their life potential. He is the founder of Body-Centered Leadership.

Dr. Amy Albright is a doctor of acupuncture and Chinese medicine and has been practicing acupressure on babies and children for over twenty years. She has a twelve-year-old son whose childhood discomforts have been avoided or reduced by using the techniques she has offered in this book.

The BeatBuds are an interactive and educational music act that children and parents love dearly. Look out for their new animated show on Nickelodeon!

Dr. Matthew Bernstein is an L.A.-based doctor of chiropractic. A father of four, Dr. Bernstein specializes in pediatrics and understands the many parents who turn to his practice for education and relief.

Dr. Robert Hamilton is a Santa Monica–based pediatrician with over thirty years of practice, FAAP (fellow of the American Academy of Pediatrics), and founder of Pacific Ocean Pediatrics. Dr. Hamilton was made famous for his YouTube video of "The Hold," a unique technique he developed to calm a crying baby.

Lisa Eberly Mastela, MPH, RD, is a registered dietitian nutritionist and a mom, with experience in nutrition counseling with children with cystic fibrosis, children on the autism spectrum, and children with feeding complications who were formerly preterm. She is the founder and CEO of Bumpin Blends, which helps support the nutrition needs of expecting and new mothers.

Melanie Wattles, RN, is a registered nurse with over twenty-five years of experience in pediatric and neonatal nursing. Melanie is also a Certified Infant Massage Instructor (CIMI 1&2) and a Certified Pediatric Massage Therapist (CPMT). Melanie owns Baby Strokes, an Austin, Texas–based massage instruction school. Melanie received her CIMI certification through the International Association of Infant Massage and CIMI2 through WINC: World Institute for Nurturing Communication.

acknowledgments

To our fantastic agent, Steve Troha, thank you for always encouraging and supporting our lunatic endeavors. This book would not be here without you. Thank you also to Kat Odom-Tomchin and the Folio Literary Management team.

A huge helping of gratitude to our incredible editor, Nina Shield, who championed our creativity, amplified our voice, and believed in this project from the start. Many thanks to the TarcherPerigee team for bringing your tremendous talents to this project. This includes but certainly is not limited to Marian Lizzi, Megan Newman, Hannah Steigmeyer, Alex Casement, and Carla Iannone. Hats off to the great art and design team: Laura Palese, Jess Morphew, Lorie Pagnozzi, Katy Riegel, Anne Chan, and Paul Girard. Thank you all over and over again!

A special thank-you from the bottom of our hearts to Amy Jindra and Nick Schlavensky, who are not only brilliant artists but also an absolute joy to work with.

And to all our friends; the moms and dads who continue to share the journey of becoming parents with us. Through the blowouts and blowups, we treasure getting to grow up with you and yours.